The psychology of person identification

The psychology of person identification

Brian R. Clifford

and

Ray Bull

North East London Polytechnic

Routledge & Kegan Paul
London, Henley and Boston

First published in 1978
by Routledge & Kegan Paul Ltd
39 Store Street,
London WC1E 7DD,
Broadway House,
Newtown Road,
Henley-on-Thames,
Oxon RG9 1EN and
9 Park Street,
Boston, Mass. 02108, USA
Set in 11 on 12 point Old Style Series 2
and Printed in Great Britain by
Lowe & Brydone

British Library Cataloguing in Publication Data

Clifford, Brian R

  The psychology of person identification.
  1. Social perception   2. Identification
  I. Title   II. Bull, Ray
  153.7'5   HM132   78-40107

ISBN 0-7100-8867-1

This book is dedicated to those with whom
we identify
C., J., S., J., E., and H.

Contents

By human goodness is meant not fineness of physique, but a right condition of the psyche. That being so, it is evident that the statesman ought to have some inkling of psychology.

Aristotle, *Nichomachean Ethics*

Preface

The question of person identification is a topic which has generated much heat but very little light in the last few years. This is the first book which looks at the problem from a specifically psychological perspective. We believe that in this psycholegal area psychology already possesses the theory and method to make important practical and theoretical contributions to the ongoing debate. Contrary to the common-sense belief that person identification is a simple affair we will be concerned to map out just how difficult recognition of a once-seen person really is, and most of the extant literature pertaining to person recognition is reviewed, described and discussed to make this point.

The difficulty of person identification resides in the fact that such identification is multidetermined. The accuracy of a witness is a complex function of social, situational and individual factors which often are not easily discernible in real-life criminal episodes but which do become tractable within the confines of a 'laboratory' experiment where they can either be controlled, partialled out, or manipulated and taken direct account of. This type of experimental approach is a very necessary first step along the road to policy recommendations concerning this thorny area of legal justice.

In the social aspects of person identification we discuss internal social attitudes, beliefs and values, especially stereotypes and how they enter into the supposed perceptual-memory aspects of viewing and remembering persons. Over and above these internalized social dimensions we also point out how the external social situation can markedly alter the accuracy of recall for a seen person or event. Such social aspects as other witnesses, and police officers trying to elicit statements and descriptions, are discussed. Other witnesses can create conformity effects in a testimony which produce consensus in error, while police officers if not very careful can insinuate distortions in visual memory by their verbal questions. The social aspects of person recognition, both internal and external, are nowhere better evidenced than in identification parades. Here these two aspects, together with specifically cognitive processes, coalesce to produce some very 'odd' behaviour, which we investigate. Our investigations lead us to suggest some radical surgery in the way identification parades are conducted.

The situational aspects which crucially determine eyewitness reliability are such things as the nature of the crime – a rape seems to be qualitatively different from a robbery – the length of exposure to the criminal, and the situation of viewing, whether bystander or victim. We evaluate the evidence, where it exists, of the effect of these and other aspects of the 'criminal' situation.

Individual factors are perhaps the most important considerations in understanding person identification, and yet they are the most difficult to assess. We attempt to show how perception and memory are selective and decision-making processes, and as such are prone to error, and this is true for all people. Man is neither a tape recorder nor a camera. People do differ, however, in other crucially important ways. Thus we look at individual differences, as they relate to person identification, in for example age, sex, suggestibility, imagery ability, cognitive style and personality, and we compare policemen and civilians as two groups of people who may differ in their ability to process and store an image of a seen person.

While evaluation of reliability by interested parties requires knowledge of these three main factors, other information is also necessary. Is it still possible, and admissible, to identify a person as a criminal if his face was never seen? The basic means of recognition is by face, and this is reflected in our book, but other means are possible. Two such identificatory modes are voice and gait. The accrued knowledge concerning these potential modes of identification is documented and where gaps still exist these are made explicit.

Another whole area which requires clarification is the means whereby police officers can best achieve correct recognition and recall. We evaluate the identification parade procedure and the efficacy of the photo-fit construction, and the allied techniques of artist's impressions, and their attendant problems. We also explore the growing area of man-machine interaction which could represent a fundamental advance in person recognition.

We are aware that psychologists often create more problems than they solve, but only by making interested bodies aware of the 'state of the art' can we lay down a sound foundation upon which future psycho-legal reciprocity can flourish. Throughout the book our aim is at least three-fold: to educate the public (as future witnesses or jurors) in the matter of person identification; to inform the judiciary of the factors that need to be weighed if the scales of justice are to be stabilized initially; and finally to crystallize and point to future research areas for psychologists who would like to feel that they are working in a meaningful field of human behaviour.

The informal contacts we have made while writing this book are too numerous to detail but we would like to thank Bob Buckhout and Alvin Goldstein for making available to us a large amount of unpublished work. Also we should like to thank Hadyn Ellis, Graham Davies and John Shepherd for availing us of their as yet unpublished researches into photo-fit.

We would like finally to acknowledge all the secretarial help we received from Janet, Lillian and Mary, who did not flinch or lose their good humour as each new illegible draft was placed before them.

1 Introduction

One of the main reasons for this book being written was the desire on the part of many organizations, groups and individuals to be cognizant of the factors which influence our identification and recognition of other people. In May 1974 in response to general disquiet the Home Secretary appointed Lord Devlin to chair a committee to examine the law and procedures on identification. The former chief of the Metropolitan Police, Sir Robert Mark, is quoted as saying that, 'If the police, the lawyers and the courts did their jobs properly the most likely cause of wrongful conviction is mistaken identity', and Lord Gardiner that, 'Most wrong convictions were on the matter of identification' (Cole and Pringle, 1974). If such statements are valid then not only may an innocent person be found guilty, but the true culprit could still be at large. However, to decide whether these views have any validity is a very difficult problem indeed. There are, of course, one or two cases in which incorrect recognition has played a part, but to determine how widespread such a phenomenon is seems almost impossible. Nevertheless, some people claim that, 'There is certainly a persuasive argument that the human memory for faces is so fallible that evidence of identification is virtually worthless. It seems likely that most people are quite incapable of remembering a face' (Cole and Pringle, 1974). Upon examination it appears that these views are based on what amounts to anecdotal evidence. Now anecdotal evidence may

I

eventually be proved correct, but until it is, it cannot serve to inform the debates on either identification evidence or on potential changes in judicial procedure. We might ask then to what extent methodologically rigorous studies have investigated our powers of person identification. This book is an attempt to present the psychological information that is presently available concerning this question.

Marshall (1969) believes that, 'The life of our courts, the trial process, is based upon the fiction that witnesses see and hear correctly and so testify; and if they do not testify with accuracy on direct examination, cross-examination will straighten them out.' This (latter) 'is another fiction.' The credibility of an eyewitness is a matter of fact for the jury to determine, but in the past, and to a very large extent still today, jurors and potential jurors do not regard eyewitness identification with scepticism. The concept of identification as it is used by the legal profession seems to imply that perception and memory, as it operates in person identification, is a simple single process, and thus if we can assume suitable conditions of viewing and no mental abnormality then failure to recall or recognize is simply a case of wilfulness or lack of probity. This simplistic view of person identification is one we will be very concerned to deny. Person identification in a criminal situation will be argued to be at least a three-stage process. The first stage involves witnessing the incident and thus involves perception and all its vagaries. The second stage involves either recounting the person's appearance to the police, trying to construct a photo-fit or attempting to aid a police artist in creating a 'likeness' of the seen criminal and all these procedures involve memory and its inherent fallibilities. The third stage sees memory and perception operating in tandem when the witness either tries to locate the criminal in a photo album of criminals, or when he tries to match current perceptions of line-up paraders to his or her stored image of the seen criminal. The important point to stress is that error can creep in at any and all of these three stages.

As such then we take for granted, and will not be concerned to laboriously document, Kubie's (1959) assertion that people quite often do not see or hear things which are presented clearly to their senses, but do 'see' and 'hear' things which are not there, and further that people frequently do not remember things which happened to them but do remember things which did not happen to them.

While we accept the fact of fallibility in eyewitness testimony we will try to explain why this phenomenon occurs, and how remediation may be inaugurated. The reason why we can accept the facts of fallibility so easily is that they have been replicated many times in the experimental literature. The psychology of testimony has a long history and in fact was one of the first areas of applied psychology, although at that time it tended to be descriptive and programmatic rather than explanatory.

The most important source of early literature on forensic and general psychology was the annual reviews provided by Whipple between 1910 and 1917. The opening shot was fired by Freud in 1906 when he argued that psychologists should be used to ascertain the truth or otherwise of a testimony. This was taken up by Munsterberg in 1908 in the USA in his book *On the Witness Stand* where he stressed the need for legal reform based upon scientific experimentation. This call was reiterated by a German criminologist Gross (1911) and together they served to spawn a great deal of appropriate work which drove home the point that sense data were fallible, recall was idiosyncratic and eyewitness testimony was inherently unreliable. The academic psychologists were also very much involved in this forensically stimulated research area (this is best seen in the work of Binet (1897) and Stern (1903–38)). Binet investigated visual memory for pictures and this work was of at least indirect relevance to identification evidence. He showed clearly that observer factors contribute more than stimulus factors. Stern built upon this visual work but went beyond it by evolving the 'event', 'reality' or 'simulated crime' experiment. 'His experiment, demonstrating unreliability in recall for unexpected events, has become the paradigm for subsequent experimental studies of eyewitness reports by both psychologists and lawyers' (Levine and Tapp, 1973). The 'event' experiment was re-employed by Kobler (1915) and by Marston (1924), and has been developed by Buckhout (e.g. 1974b) and Loftus (e.g. 1975) in America, and by the Psychology Departments of the North East London Polytechnic and Nottingham University in England.

The fruitful reciprocity between law and psychology is best seen in the work of Hutchins and Slesinger (1928), the first a lawyer and the second a psychologist. They reviewed legal rules of evidence in terms of psychological findings on perception, memory and emotion, ultimately arguing for a still greater effort in interdisciplinary experimentation and application. This clarion call was echoed by Gardner, a lawyer, in 1933, who himself outlined positive lines of advance for future research. Two other treatises on legal psychology ought to be mentioned; McCarty (1929) and Burtt (1931) systematically related the role of such psychological parameters as stress, emotion and attention to perception and memory as they operated in a legal setting and verified experimentally the unreliability of identification. The later books by Wall (1965) and Marshall (1966) were designed for the legal profession and unfortunately were somewhat light on sustained experimental evidence. Marshall succeeds in showing, by his own research using a staged incident, that social classes differ in the content of their recalls, that police are somewhat different from civilians in the amount and type of evidence they offered as testimony, and that we must be aware of the selective processes of perception and memory and the 'inventive reconstructions' of witnesses, together with the internal gambling procedures of witnesses at line-ups.

Hopefully, this potted history of classical studies will serve to show both an intimate interaction between forensic and general psychology, the possibility of extrapolation from pure to applied research in memory and perception and the application and elucidation of insights already existing in psychology to the area of identification evidence. This book is intended to build on these earlier studies and to try and explain why these documented fallibilities in identification occur.

Devlin (1976) called for exploration, of a research nature, into 'establishing ways in which the insights of psychology could be brought to bear on the conduct of identification parades and the practice of the courts in all matters relating to evidence of identification' (p.73). This has been a fundamental orientation of the present book, and is reflected in most of the chapters but especially the first two, where the insights we look at are those gleaned from research into cognitive processes and research of a more psycho-social nature.

Following Neisser (1967), cognitive psychology can be characterized as those branches of psychological research which deal with complex perception, the organization of memory, language, thinking and, most generally, man's intellectual processes.

Like all science, psychology has employed a number of general and specific simplifying assumptions and procedures. One such general simplifying procedure was to treat perception, memory, thinking, problem-solving and language as separate and separable processes. The reasons for breaking down, or of dividing up, the human being have been couched in terms of 'heuristic usefulness', 'experimental expediency' or simply 'manageability'. However, such devices have an unsavoury habit of becoming first conceptual distinctions and then ontological realities. Thus in the end one can glibly talk about 'laws of memory' which are unqualified by such factors as the role of language, thinking, valuing, believing or feeling.

Over and above the incapacitating outcome of the above general simplifying assumptions other more specific ways of conducting research arose which prevented the possibility of the direct application of experimental findings to the judicial process. These more specific simplifying procedures were concerned with the choice of theoretical models with which to interpret the data, and in the conception of man from which these interpreting theories were derived.

The theoretical models of man with which experimental psychology operates are noteworthy both for their dissimilarity one from the other and for their common dissimilarity with the reality which exists when a person sees a criminal episode and tries to remember it (and the chief criminal figures) for later reconstruction for the police. The models which were tried and failed were man as a black box, man as a telephone switch-board and man as a computer. All these failed for a greater or lesser number of reasons, but all were inadequate uniformly because they failed to take into account man's thinking, feeling, believing totality.

This last point leads into the single most damaging feature of psychology's intellectual history. Our conception of man's nature has hampered development in both pure and applied research. Behaviourism was the heir to associationism and in turn left a legacy to memory research which stipulated that the memorizer was essentially a passive recipient rather than an active perceiver, conceiver and memorizer. He was regarded as passive in the sense of contributing nothing to the input in terms of pre-existing knowledge, perhaps because he was a black box, and he was seen as contributing nothing to the encoding, storage, and rearrangement of memories, perhaps because perception was judged to be like a camera and memory like a tape recorder or videotape.

To a large extent the influence of these theoretical biases in psychology's history can be seen in the methodological decisions it made. Ebbinghaus (1885) can be viewed as the founding father of experimental memory research, and he wished to study the 'pure processes of memory' uncontaminated by everyday habits of thought and experience. As a result of this wish, and influenced by the pre-theoretical assumptions described above, the vast literature in early memory research was composed almost entirely of memory for nonsense material, especially the consonant-vowel-consonant trigram (CVC). The power of implicit assumptions about man and the progress of science can be seen clearly here. While Ebbinghaus was aware of the possible inter-relationship between cognitive sub-processes he none the less fell foul of the general simplifying assumption that they could be separated. His use of nonsense syllables was the monumental error which misguided future psychology for nearly three quarters of a century, and indirectly rendered law enforcement agencies poverty-stricken in terms of a scientific basis for the execution of their duties. In terms of person identification Ebbinghaus, and especially his tradition, was doubly crippling because it used material devoid of meaning, and he used only verbal material. It can legitimately be argued that Ebbinghaus could not do everything at once, and this would be conceded, but it cannot be accepted that hundreds upon hundreds of psychologists should have slavishly followed his methodology and used his material to the exclusion of all else, never asking themselves questions about generality and applicability. Jenkins (1974) captures the tenor of this argument when he says that Ebbinghaus committed a particularly disastrous error, and goes on to say that his method, his material and his own orientation combine to hide the otherwise overwhelming effect of knowledge which is the most powerful variable in memorization. If one studies any effect after first removing the chief source of variance one will get the most odd results. We will see this clearly in terms of meaning, and factors over and above meaning, when we compare identification of people in the laboratory with identification of people in more real-life situations, where it will be shown that performance drops markedly in the latter.

Fortunately for an applied psychology of memory the edifice of theoretical error and the mist of misbegotten facts are now beginning to be demolished and dispersed, and we can but hope that the 'cultural lag' between the practical help we can offer those who have to deal with psychological phenomena in practice and the institutions of psychological research will not be too protracted. It will be some time but the future looks decidedly brighter. The theoretical tide began to turn about the 1960s, although it was charted as early as 1932 with the, now realized, futuristic work of Bartlett. The watershed was the publication in 1967 of a book called *Cognitive Psychology* by Ulric Neisser. The cognitive approach to human functioning refers to the study of all the processes by which the sensory input is transformed, reduced, elaborated, stored, recovered and used. As such it recognizes that perception, language, thinking and problem-solving are intimately interconnected, and must be given full consideration in any one field of interest, such as person identification. All these processes must be considered in a full and adequate explanation of eyewitness recognition.

Thus, at a stroke cognitive psychology overcame the first general simplifying procedure of decoupling the memory system from all the other subsystems. It also stressed the active subject and the fallacy of a black box approach. Most cognitive psychologists pay at least lip service to the fact of emotion and man's connotative being, but very little research has manipulated these as possible important considerations. This, however, is basically a residual problem based on, and largely a function of, the fact that most research has been carried out in the laboratory. It will only be a matter of time before such factors are being routinely explored. We will see from experiments which use more real-life situations, from our own studies at the North East London Polytechnic, and from court cases, that many cognitive phenomena associated with person identification are incomprehensible unless one takes into account what the person is, what he is trying to do, and the way his beliefs, values and motivations act not only at the time of perception but also during the period of storage and especially at the time of recall or recognition.

The second set of insights which we explore in terms of person identification are those found within social psychology. While we are concerned to stress that perception and memory are selective and interpretative we also want to go beyond this by postulating that these systems are at base social systems. The mechanisms of perception and memory are indistinguishable and inseparable from man as a social being. Person identification is customarily carried out in a social context, thus an adequate analysis of the topic requires that the eyewitness be viewed from a social-psychological perspective. An understanding of perception, memory and decision-making in identification situations involves considering such things as stereotyping, prejudice, implicit personality theorizing, and conformity to others, together with an appreciation of personality needs, social values, expectancies and evaluative apprehensiveness. Some of these 'insights' are discussed at length in this book, others more tangentially.

A few words should perhaps be said about the type of literature we will be discussing and analysing. Throughout the book we will draw on evidence which is both directly and indirectly relevant to the specific question of person identification. This we believe to be legitimate because while stimulus material may differ (for example, words can be presented auditorially or visually, objects can be presented themselves or as pictures, and faces can be presented either 'live' or in the form of photographs), the basic processes of memory are the same, at least qualitatively and should at the very least offer speculative predictions as to what would happen in real-life situations of criminal episodes, and later recognition of the criminal. We will thus draw liberally upon 'laboratory' studies which look at memory for faces presented as photographs and pointedly compare estimates of man's ability to recognize a seen face from these studies with estimates of the same ability obtained under 'mock crime' situations where actual people are seen perpetrating a crime and are then re-presented for identification. We will quickly see that these two estimates differ markedly. Thus, throughout we will be concerned to indicate, describe and draw inferences from extant research which we believe is relevant and transferable to, but not directly derived from, actual real-life person recognition or identification. This may limit the validity of our conclusions and render our judgments susceptible to refinement and modification in the light of future, more applied, research undertakings. A question which exercised us greatly was whether we were writing this book too soon but we are of the opinion that the current status of psychological theory and factual knowledge is sufficiently developed to warrant this volume. Not only are rich insights and relevant researches now available but some guidelines for future research are badly needed. Over and above the state of psychological research there is also the need of the judiciary to have at their fingertips an up-to-date and comprehensive review of current findings in person identification if the letter and spirit of the Devlin Report is to be executed. Chapter 2 thus looks at the new approach to memory and perception, and then goes on to argue that while apparently quantitatively superior, visual memory is at base no different from verbal memory and both are concerned with extracting meaning from the various inputs. We next compare visual memory for facial and non-facial material and argue that, once again, we need postulate no separate processes for the two systems. As a precursor to Chapter 4 we summarize the evidence which shows excellent memory of faces presented as photographs, but immediately counsel caution in using these estimates to argue that person identification is not a problem by presenting evidence from 'simulated crime' studies which give very much lower estimates of man's ability to remember and recognize a seen face. These latter studies strongly suggest that unexpectedness, brevity of exposure and stress are three of the many factors which are necessary considerations in understanding and evaluating eyewitness testimony, over and above the inherent limitations of man's perceptual and memorial ability.

Chapter 3 examines the possibility that witnesses may have stereotypic expectancies and notions about the kinds of physical appearance they expect criminals to have. It is argued that such stereotypes may play a role in person identification especially when confabulation occurs because memory is inefficient. It will be shown that contrary to the belief of many pundits a member of the general public may well have powerful expectancies about the appearance of criminals. If you glimpsed a mugger briefly would you on an identification parade be inclined to pick out someone who was young and scruffy or someone more mature – dressed in a smart suit?

Chapter 4 looks at the chief source of identification – identification by means of face. In this chapter we look at recognition of seen faces (from photographic presentation and real-life crime episodes) and at recall, as measured by photo-fit construction. In so doing we outline what is currently known about facial scanning patterns, what features are most salient for later recognition, whether single features, features in combination or attributes are most important for identification, and then relate these to the actual practice of photo-fit construction as expressed by a recent Home Office survey. Once again we compare real-life recognition with recognition levels found in the laboratory and indicate the differences, and hopefully, their causes. We conclude the chapter by looking at man-machine recognition devices.

Chapter 5 looks at person identification by means other than by face, especially voice. A crime seldom takes place in silence. Usually the criminal issues instructions or demands some sort of obedience. Just how good memory is for a person's voice, how much of a speech sample we must hear, whether memory for a voice shows the same decrease over time as does visual memory are questions which this chapter addresses.

We then, in Chapter 6, pick up that thread of cognitive psychology again which suggests that we cannot separate visual memory from verbal memory. Specifically we look at the role of labelling by the witness, and questioning by the 'interrogator' as potential sources of enhancement or detraction of reliable memory for a seen person or event. We show that our memories can be aided by the use of language but also that we can seriously 'bewitch' witnesses by the questions we ask, and the way we ask them.

Chapter 7 looks at individual and group differences in eyewitness reliability. Such differences have a long history in psychology. Children's imagination and suggestibility are well known, but two possible views are explored – one which says children should make poor witnesses, the other which makes the opposite prediction. Levine and Tapp (1971) conducted an informal interview with a large police force and found that they seemed to prefer female witnesses to male. We review the evidence of male and female differences in identification accuracy and make the case that it may depend upon the sex of the seen person and the nature of the criminal episode. Other factors investigated in this chapter include personality differences (such as need for affiliation, need for approval, introversion and extroversion), individual differences in imagery ability, and in cognitive style. We end the chapter by comparing police and civilians as eye-witnesses. Throughout this chapter we try to suggest possible screening devices for law enforcement agencies which could perhaps give some suggestion as to who is a good witness.

Chapter 8 tackles the thorny issue of identification parades. We suggest a number of alternatives to that used in England at the present time, and focus our chapter on the cognitive and social aspects of identification in this situation. Sources of bias are discussed in the light of these insights, and remedies are tentatively suggested. We are aware that by 'tightening up' identification parades we may be contributing to the miscarriage of justice by implanting in the minds of jurors the belief that because the identification parade is 'now perfect' any positive identification must be correct and accurate. However, if the underlying message of this book is absorbed – to educate all potential victims, jurors and eyewitnesses in the what and how of person identification – this potential damage should be nullified.

Our concluding chapter 'Retrospect and Prospect', seeks to show why psychology has not been regarded as very helpful to police forces and the judiciary in the past and to show how it could, in the future, be not only helpful but also seen to be helpful. Throughout the book we suggest that one of the reasons why psychology has not to date contributed much to the debate on identification is the fact that most psychologists have become very specialized in one or two particular areas. This book is an attempt to redress the balance and to show how several approaches to the study of behaviour can be combined to give a clearer picture of what actually takes place. The study of person identification is a growing area with, however, an intrinsic dilemma based on methodological paradigms. Many of the findings confirm that, 'Acquisitions of discriminations among human faces, complex and infinitely variable as faces are, can be said to be one of the truly staggering feats of perceptual learning of which human beings are capable' (Chance, Goldstein and Schicht, 1967). Shepherd and Ellis (1973) also emphasize the point that faces are better recognized than almost any other form of visual stimulus material ever investigated. However, when we look at the evidence from simulated crime experimentation quite the opposite conclusion is driven. The statements of Chance *et al.* and Shepherd and Ellis are based on data gathered in the laboratory where, first, the observer usually has a fairly long while to look at each stimulus and, second, there is a very meaningful difference from the real world in emotional atmosphere. In the laboratory the subject has little else to focus his attention on but the experimental stimuli and these are typically static photographs rather than a person in motion. Here everything is conducive to high performance and there is little emotional stress, which we now know not only narrows attention but also results in rather simplistic and crude perceptual processes being employed. Further it is possible, as Freud suggested, that unpleasant experiences are most difficult to recall and as Edwards (1941) notes, recall is poorest for those factors 'which are not in harmony with an individual's existing frame of reference'. Penry (1971) points out that real-life witnesses are often required to describe 'a face which has come out of the blue and disappeared with the same suddenness leaving an aftermath of confusion, fear or shock'. Similarly on 11 May 1975 the *Observer* stated that, 'A conviction that rests in the last analysis on a witness's recall over a period of weeks or months of a face seen fleetingly at the moment of high tension appears to be basically unsafe.' What seems to be needed are studies of real-life or life-like situations. One of the aims of this book is to suggest that event experimentation may be the way forward. If one can accept that such simulated crime studies approximate real-life criminal episodes better than does looking at a photographed face for later recognition then it can be seen that identification remains a problem.

In this book our overriding aim has been to raise issues, generate questions and hopefully indicate fruitful guidelines for future research, and at the same time to offer some helpful advice and factual data to law enforcement agencies so that they can better evaluate their practices and procedures. Whilst we would certainly not go so far as to say that identification evidence is usually of little value, we do believe that psychological findings can make an immense contribution in this area. However, to maximize its contribution reorientations may be necessary. The topic of identification, because it is so influenced by a *combination* of perception, memory, individual differences and social pressure (four of the corner-stones of psychology), permits, nay forces, the traditional delineations within the discipline of psychology to be crossed. Consequently, we hope that this text will enable psychologists to view some aspects of their discipline in a new light. It is not true to say that psychology can contribute little to our understanding of identification, but what is true is that no one psychologist alone has been aware of most of the relevant factors in this area. On 11 April 1976, the *Sunday Times* suggested that, 'A more radical brief than that which the Devlin Committee was given is the only approach that can significantly improve matters. The Committee was not empowered to carry out its own research and when it took evidence from experts on memory and perception most of what it heard was feeble.' We believe that the evidence which this Committee heard was as feeble as were its attempts to avail itself of much relevant psychological information. We grant that this information was spread far and wide in the literature and we have attempted to bring it all together into a single volume. In this way we hope that it will no longer be the case (as the *Sunday Times* noted in the same article) that, 'The British Legal system, and our police, are very backward in this controversial area.'

We trust that those who read this book will employ the information which it contains and therefore we shall be able to counter the criticisms that, 'Psychologists have had little impact on the law's unwarranted reliance on eye-witness reports' (Levine and Tapp, 1973). Thus, not only will this book be of value to psychologists because of its applied, cross-specialization approach to their discipline but it will also be of use to the legal profession and to all those employed in the judicial processes. Levine and Tapp (1973) further state that, 'Psychologists and lawyers both confront the problems of eye-witness evidence, but most law classrooms remain unaffected by the accrued knowledge of the mediating psychological processes.' We hope that this text will go some way towards putting this right, but we have been constantly aware that to attempt to write a book on psychology in a comprehensible yet concise way, not only for psychologists but also for the legal profession, for the police and for the public, is to attempt to balance between two stools. We have been warned that in the past books on various topics which have attempted to do this have usually failed because the layman has found them to be full of jargon and the psychologist has found them to be pedestrian. The extent to which we also have failed is for the reader to decide.

2 Cognitive aspects of person identification

INTRODUCTION

When a person is asked to reconstruct the events which took place at the scene of a crime or when he is asked to form a photo-fit construction of a seen criminal, or to identify him from amongst a number of other people in an identification parade, what basically is being assumed is that the person has perceived correctly, and what is being asked for is that the person use his memory. Thus the psychology of perception and memory, which has been well researched, ought to furnish many of the insights which the Devlin Report (1976) argued were of crucial importance if law enforcement agencies were to prosecute justice better in the sense of apprehending the guilty and excusing the innocent.

The insights contained within cognitive psychology stress that witnesses are active and selective, who, at the point of perception, search through the outside world and select from it, then make decisions about what to store and how to store it. These decision processes are informed and directed by already existing spatial, logical and pragmatic knowledge structures. Depending upon the total situation, the perceiver employs different storage formats of what he has seen and often quite unconsciously he will encode information in more than one format. Irrespective of storage format the overriding aim will be to assimilate perceived events to existing knowledge and beliefs, in order to avoid discrepancies with what he knows about causality, people and things.

This view of how humans process information in general and how eyewitnesses go about perceiving, recognizing or identifying a seen person in particular has vital implications for testimony. Thus, as Buckhout (1974b) indicates, when a person is asked to identify someone he or she is being asked to do something that the normal human was not created to do.[Human memory and perception are selective and decision-making processes, which function to create sense out of chaotic experience, and not to produce reliable eyewitness testimony. The thesis to be developed in this chapter is that memory is constructive and reconstructive using existing epistemic structures or existing knowledge as a reference or base. To view perception and memory as copying processes is entirely wrong and very dangerous. [Juries must be aware of this in the future and the weight carried by eyewitness testimony must be re-evaluated. Like scientists, jurors have models, analogies or metaphors of what the human being is like. Unfortunately, the prevailing models are that men perceive visually like a videotape, and remember auditorially like a tape recorder. A tape suffers from no interference because, once stored, memories move along and a fresh storage location is made available and these different locations are not in connection with one another. Also a tape allows of no decay because once established it is always there and, because always there, no retrieval problems ensue, it is simply a matter of time till the right storage location is found. Man, his perception and his memory are just not like that. Just what they are like will now be discussed, perception briefly, memory more extensively.

PERCEPTION AND ATTENTION

It has been customary in experimental psychology to separate perceptual and memorial processes, but to a large extent these are inseparable. One perceives in terms of stored categories; these categories being built up from previously perceived regularities. Memory for events requires that these events were actually perceived: the testing of perception after the disappearance of the perceived object necessarily requires a consideration of memory.

Research, and a little reflection, show that perception is fallible – why should this be? One reason is that perception is limited. It is not limited so much in terms of actual registration but rather in the conversion of these sensory inputs into more durable formats for memory (e.g. Sperling, 1960, 1967). This is the so-called encoding problem. The best evidence for this limitation is the work by Potter (1976; Potter and Levy, 1969), at least with complex material. She presents evidence that a picture of a scene can be recognized, that is, processed and matched to an internal representation, within one eighth of a second but that a further one third of a second is required for storage of that scene in memory. If this further time is not available, or is not utilized for encoding, then no memory remains of what has been seen. A vitally important question here is whether the encoding of visual input is achieved by verbal means or whether visual input is encoded in visual form for storage and retention, irrespective of the form of testing. This question will exercise us greatly in the section on memory but to anticipate slightly it will be argued that the relationship between the encoding dimension (visual or verbal) and the testing situation (identification parade, photo-fit or verbal description) is absolutely crucial.

Another reason for the fallibility of perception is that perception is selective. Because we cannot encode all we register in conditions of information overload a selection mechanism must come into operation. This mechanism is primed by what is already in the mind of the perceiver. Perceptions are not directly given, rather one learns to perceive, and to perceive selectively. Perceptual processing involves organizing discrete elements of a situation into meaningful categories and wholes. Pre-existing categories will vary from one individual to the next, because of his upbringing. Thus different people will selectively attend to different aspects of an event, person or place. We will look more closely at this when we investigate inter-racial differences in recognition of own and other races, and we will also make the case that the existence of face stereotypes, situation stereotypes and event stereotypes are similarly based upon the interaction of perceptual strategies and stored categories. As Bruner (1958) put it so succinctly, 'the . . . organism has a highly limited span of attention, and a highly limited span of immediate memory. [thus] Selectivity is forced upon us by the nature of these limitations.'

Inherent limitations and psychologically generated selectivity lead to the third reason for poor perception: perceptual confabulation. Since we can only register a fraction of the possible input, and code only a fraction of that, we are left with gaps. These gaps are filled by 'appropriate' material in order to render the observations coherent. This 'filling in' process which goes on unconsciously, and hence cannot be detected or eradicated, is usually achieved by means of inferences which serve to combine the authentic (perceived) fragments into a chain of events which is logically understandable. This mechanism of logical and psychological completion cannot be stressed too strongly.

Inadequate attention deployment is another source of poor perception. The more attention one allocates to an object or event the more chance there is of actually seeing relevant features. In laboratory research attention deployment is likely to be maximally efficient with the attendant possibility of very high recognition scores when memory is later tested. In real-life criminal episodes, however, a victim may concentrate all his attention on aspects of the situation relevant to escape, rather than stimuli concerned with the appearance of the criminal. We should be careful of equating duration of criminal episode with probability of eyewitness identification. In threatening situations victims and bystanders will most likely be engaged in diffuse anxiety reactions which are maximally defective for later person recognition. Emotion has a disorganizing effect on both perception and memory. Kobler (cited in Whipple, 1915) concluded, at the end of a real-life study, that excitement and emotion affect observational ability. Beier (1952) in the same vein showed that anxiety caused loss of abstract ability generally and a loss of flexibility in intellectual functioning and visual perception. Berrien (1955) argued that excitement blurs accuracy and subsequent reporting of criminal events, and Buckhout (1974b) reported that air crews progressively decreased monitoring of instruments as anxiety increased. We will also show later, from our own studies, that anxiety or arousal interacts complexly with the sex and personality of the witness.

Over and above these psychological facets of perception it is also the case that people differ in perceptual capacity due to sensory deficits. Such defects are probably more numerous than the wearing of glasses and hearing aids would suggest. A fundamental requirement of a reliable eyewitness is that their sense organs be functionally adequate. Industrial noise has greatly increased the number of people who are functionally deaf, and medical sources suggest that about 4 per cent of males and 1 per cent of females are colour blind. Short and long sightedness would seem to be obvious considerations in the evaluation of eyewitness reliability.

Given these numerous influences on perception we should not be too surprised when Buckhout (1975a) indicates, with hard data, that nearly 2,000 witnesses can be wrong in selecting, from a line-up, the person seen mugging a woman a few seconds earlier and who then ran face forward into a TV camera. This would be predicted from a knowledge of sensory malfunctioning, limited perceptual capacity, selectivity, encoding styles, logical filling in and pre-existing categories, together with the influence of set and attention, and the difficulty in the sudden situation of criminal episodes. These factors would help explain poor eyewitness reliability but there is yet another factor – memory – which is a crucial consideration in person identification given that we can assume adequate perception took place. It is to this we now turn.

MEMORY RESEARCH AND ITS APPLICATION

Measurement of memory

Before we discuss the type of situation used in the laboratory to test how good or bad memory is, and before we look at the various theories which have been used to explain why memory is far from perfect, it is necessary to examine the variety of methods used to measure memory performance, and to look at how closely they approximate the situations used in police procedures.

Memory has been traditionally measured in a number of ways but for our purposes they can be broadly divided into two: recall and recognition.

Recall

Recall is a measure of retention in which no external help is given to the recaller in his attempt to retell what he saw or heard.

This is analogous to the type of memory being asked for when a policeman asks the witness, 'Can you describe the man you saw running away from the car?' Within the general category of 'recall', techniques of 'cued recall' have been used. This is similar to the case where the police ask, 'Can you describe the colour of the person's hair, the colour of his trousers?', or where, in a photo-fit construction, the officer 'starts the witness off' with, say, a round-shaped chin or head shape, after the witness has furnished the descriptive label 'round'. From this visual cue the witness recalls that it was 'not so round' or 'much rounder', etc. These visual cues trigger off other remembered features.

Over and above these two highly researched measures of memory performance which, it has been argued, have direct parallels in police procedure there is a third method of eliciting remembered events which, while increasingly coming under police scrutiny, has been almost totally neglected by psychologists. Most research in recall and cued recall memory have used experimental material provided by the experimenter, and tested memory while the subject has been fully conscious. There is, however, another approach to recall which tests memory for non-experimental material and which deliberately employs non-conscious subjects. The type of memory being probed is usually referred to as re-dintegrative memory, where the memories are often of things long past, for example, childhood experiences. One reason why psychologists have not used this approach to examine memory for personal autobiography is the lack of a check on the reality of the remembered events. Another reason is that in most cases such memories have been elicited by special techniques such as hypnosis. Notwithstanding psychology's reluctance to accept this technique in experimentation, Reiff and Scheerer (1959) showed that adult memories for schoolroom experiences are greater under hypnosis than during fully awake conscious recall. The recalled events in this case could be independently verified. Recently, a great deal of interest has been raised by the success of the Israeli police with the use of hypnosis in criminal cases. There is no doubt that they lead the world in this technique. So efficient are they that in one year seventeen arrests have been made, directly ascribable to the use of hypnosis. One outstanding case was that of a bus driver who was involved in a terrorist bombing of his bus. All the driver could remember was that a man got on the bus at a stop, with a parcel. Under hypnosis he was able to help construct an identikit picture of a man so life-like that the second person it was shown to was able to put a name to the face. The terrorist was caught and confessed to the crime.

The American police are latching on to this new method of eliciting eyewitness testimony. The Californian Police Department used hypnosis with the 55-year-old driver of the school bus which was kidnapped with all twenty-six children on board. When interviewed by the police at the time of the crime he could remember little about the vans used by the three criminals to transport the children from the bus to the underground hideout. However, under hypnosis he provided a vital clue – the last five letters and digits of one of the van's number plate. The New Jersey Force have also employed hypnosis beneficially. A patrol man who witnessed the death of a 69-year-old man in a hit-and-run incident could not remember the number of the car. Under hypnosis he recalled four of the six numbers. The criminals were eventually arrested.

Britain has regrettably been rather slow in investigating the possible use of hypnosis in criminal cases. Only a few instances have been recorded. One such case involved Dr Lionel Haward of the Psychology Department of the University of Surrey. The police were anxious to trace a man who had been seen walking along a platform by a woman who had discovered a body on a train. This man could have been the murderer but the woman was unable to furnish an adequate description. Dr Haward placed the woman under hypnosis and was able to elicit a 1,000-word description of the person she had seen. The man was traced, and found to be innocent. His presence on the platform had been purely coincidental but by eliminating him a great saving in police man-hours was achieved. It is often forgotten that eyewitness testimony operates not only to identify suspects but also to eliminate them. While a great many safeguards have to be inaugurated, both ethical and scientific, none the less the use of hypnosis as a means of probing eyewitness testimony should be rigorously investigated. It follows from our discussion of perception that, because more information is registered sensorially than is encoded for conscious memory, it is possible that the input is stored, some in easily accessible format, some not so accessible. It may be the latter type of material that requires hypnosis to allow access.

Recognition

Recognition memory is involved when the initial stimulus is re-presented and the person simply has to express a feeling of familiarity. This is the case in identification parades when the criminal, if in custody, is presented and the witness, if he remembers him, simply has to say, 'Yes that is he'. Current memory research is divided as to whether recognition is, in fact, as simple as this. Some theorists argue that recognition merely involves a one-stage decision process as to the familiarity of the to-be-identified stimulus (e.g. Kintsch, 1970; Murdoch, 1968; Norman, 1968) while others argue that search and retrieval stages are as evident in recognition as in recall, i.e. that both recognition and recall are two-stage processes (e.g. Anderson and Bower, 1972; Mandler, 1972; Tulving and Thompson, 1971, 1973). As evidence for the latter view Tulving and Thompson (1973) present research findings which show recall scores to be higher than recognition – a most unusual situation in memory research. This strongly suggests that high, correct recognition at identification parades should not be assumed. This is supported by a closer look at just what recognition entails in person identification. Identification is achieved by making a comparison between a person being currently observed and a stored memory image of the original criminal. The problem of this matching process is, however, as Belbin (1956) has suggested, that the stored memory image (of the criminal) is based on features of the remembered object which are most salient or significant to the observer. That is, the witness has abstracted and coded only certain of the total possible features, and done this in ways which have been shown to be highly idiosyncratic and distorted (e.g. Bartlett, 1932). The overall problem is that where a stored memory trace and a currently perceived person only partially overlap, but do so in terms of the salient or significant features which the initial encoding produced, then there is a dramatic increase in the possibility of a false positive (wrong) identification (Levy and Heshka, 1973).

Other things being equal, however, recognition gives better

memory performance than cued recall, and cued recall gives better performance than uncued recall. The power of hypnosis as a recall technique, while apparently very great, still awaits rigorous quantification.

Theories of forgetting

Irrespective of the type of testing used all methods indicate that memory is not perfect. Psychologists have been much exercised in elucidating the process of memory fading. All memories do not fade away at the same rate, or in the same way. In the laboratory this 'curve of forgetting' is measured by testing different individuals at different time intervals since perceiving an event or learning a set of pictures or a group of items. Formerly psychologists believed that a typical curve fell rapidly at first and then gradually tapered off. However, these early studies were performed on verbal material which lacked meaning (e.g. the person was requested to retain a set of items comprising CVC (consonant-vowel-consonant) trigrams). Later experiments have shown that the curve of forgetting varies enormously with the material used and the situation of the learning. In general, meaningful material is shown to be retained much longer than nonsense material. The types of retention test used also produce different curves with recognition producing a curve that falls off much more slowly and stays at a higher level than does recall.

The question then becomes why do we forget. There are a number of possible explanations such as passive decay, systematic distortion of the memory trace, interference, retrieval failure, motivated forgetting, and displacement theories. Over and above these psychological theories, physical trauma, drug abuse and senility are other possible causes of forgetting.

The passive decay theory

This suggests that memories fade over time. Time itself cannot be an explanation but is merely the condition for supposed metabolic processes to operate to degrade the memory trace which is set up during learning or perception. While intuitively plausible there is little experimental evidence for this theory, and a good deal against it. Physical skills do not disintegrate if not practised (e.g. it is rare that anyone forgets how to ride a bike), but the main problem for passive decay theories of memory failure is that people frequently recall memories which they failed to recall at some earlier point in time.

Systematic distortion of the memory trace

It is frequently the case that a person's testimony differs markedly from his testimony about the same incident given some weeks earlier. The difference is not only in terms of quantity but also quality. Where witness testimony is available and can be checked off against the objective reality existing at the time of perception it shows recollection of events that never happened, or which were very different from the way they were reported. Processes of distortion are crucial features of human memory and we will later argue for its theoretical significance in an adequate theory of memory. A point of both theoretical and judicial importance is whether this systematic distortion of the memory trace takes place over time or at the point of initial perception. The early view of systematic distortion of the memory trace was that it went on over time. Wulf (1922) found that when subjects were presented with line drawings of simple geometrical shapes and asked to draw them at a later date the reproductions showed certain characteristic distortions when compared with the original shapes. These changes tended to be in one of three specific directions: (i) if the presented shape looked like some familiar object, the recalled shape looked even more like it; (ii) the figures became more symmetrical; (iii) any irregularity in the perceived figure became accentuated in the recalled figure. However, Hebb and Foord (1945), Riley (1962) and Bruner, Busiek and Minturn (1952) all indicate that distortions are no greater after long delays than after short delays, thus strongly implicating distortion at encoding rather than a gradual distortion over time. That distortion of memory is a very important consideration is suggested by the fact that such distortions also occur in verbal memory. New research with verbal material serves to support and clarify the earlier distortion findings of Bartlett (1932). Thorndyke (1976) shows clearly that inferences are drawn which can distort memory for connected discourse, but more importantly, that these inferences go on at input.

Where research does show systematic distortion over time is in those cases where the same subject is repeatedly tested. This can be explained by the subject remembering his own recalls (e.g. Kay, 1955). Wall (1965) provides a beautiful example of this in a court case where the witness, on repeated testimony over a number of re-trials, gives clearer and clearer descriptions of the suspect, every time she is asked. This has very serious implications for court-room procedure. Mandler and Parker (1976) have shown that 'repeated reproductions' can have a massive negative effect on the accuracy of remembered visual detail.

Interference theory of forgetting

This account of forgetting does not use time as an explanation but rather stresses that it is what we do between initial perception and later recalling that is crucial. Within this interference account of memory failure there exists interference caused by prior learning, or perception, on later learning (this is called pro-active interference, PI) and the interference caused by later learning or perception on earlier learning (this being termed retro-active interference, RI). Initial interference theories of forgetting were quite simple but recently they have become increasingly more complicated (Postman, 1972, 1976). For our purposes, however, the basic parameters are these: the more two events, scenes, places or people are alike, the more they will be confused. Similarity is a basic factor in this theory of forgetting. To take a case from real life: similarity can reside either in persons or in places. Professor Houts (cited in Wall, 1965) quotes an armed robbery case where the ticket man in a railway station was held up. The victim later picked out a sailor in a line-up as the guilty party. The sailor, however, had a good alibi and was later released. The sailor's base was near the railway station and on three separate occasions he had purchased a ticket from the ticket agent. Hout reports that when he asked the ticket agent why he had picked out the sailor in the line-up he was told 'because his face looked familiar'. He knew he had seen the face before and that they were not acquainted. Thus he assumed that

25

the familiarity related back to the robbery when in fact it undoubtedly went back to the three times he had sold the man train tickets. In this case the familiar situation had been the train station but the familiar face had been displaced from one situation to the other. This type of interference effect is often referred to as unconscious transference. The moral here is that identification is based on familiarity – something about the person identified strikes a familiar chord in the mind of the witness. Frequently, however, this familiarity is based on past experiences totally unrelated to the present crime. A witness does not simply have to pick out a suspect from an identification parade because he is familiar but because this feeling of familiarity relates directly to the criminal episode being investigated. That an interference account of memory failure is not a rarified ivory tower theory has been shown by the above case study of Wall, and as another example the first author was involved (as adviser to one of the defence counsels) in the 1976 Caribbean Club Affray Trial at the Old Bailey which lasted 109 days and cost £400,000. One crucial piece of psychological evidence was the fact that one police witness, who gave testimony and identified a suspect four weeks after the incident, had allegedly frequented the Caribbean Club in the intervening time, to monitor the coming and going of numerous coloured people. It thus seems likely that in these intervening weeks numerous sightings were made of faces which perceptually differed little from the eventually identified face. The possibility of interference effects could not be ruled out in this case. It is possible that the identified suspect had been seen at some time other than at the affray, or had been seen at the affray but not perpetrating any criminal act.

Pro-active interference has an important bearing on whether persons who have experienced coloured people frequently (because they live or work in a high immigrant area) are better at recognizing such faces than are those who do not live in a multi-racial area. There would seem to be a delicate trade-off between familiarization producing greater opportunity for learning discriminations and hence increasing perceptual and memorial powers, and familiarity producing greater interference through greater numbers of perceptual traces of 'barely distinguishable faces' being laid down in memory and which could act as potent sources of pro-active interference. This matter will be raised again when we look in Chapter 4 at face recognition of different racial groups.

Retrieval failure

It has been suggested that memories are seldom lost, they merely become inaccessible. Academic psychology makes the conceptual distinction between accessibility and availability. This is part of the reason why recall is said to be poorer than recognition. Hypnosis has suggested that if we can only find the right routes of access, memory and perception can be shown to be quite staggering in their powers. But retrieval is not the whole story: it seems as if retrieval efficiency is intimately connected and interlinked with encoding, i.e. the initial storage. Tulving and Thompson (1973) have suggested an Encoding Specificity Hypothesis of Episodic Memory. They argue that recall and recognition will be maximized when the situation of recall mirrors the situation of encoding. Context as well as specific events are encoded and become part of the memory trace and to maximize retrieval that encoded context should be reinstated at the time of recall also. Experimental studies show this clearly (e.g. Abernethy, 1940), and Hunter (1964) states that,' In general it is true to say that if the environment is greatly altered during the time of attempted remembering then remembering will be impaired.' As evidence he quotes a study where nonsense syllables were presented for learning against a coloured background and then at some later date, when forgetting had occurred, they were re-learned either against the same coloured background or a different coloured background. Against a different coloured background the second learning took much longer. The converse however does not hold: simply remembering or recognizing a person does not ensure you will remember either where you saw him or what he was doing when you saw him. Standing, Conezio and Haber (1970) presented subjects with photographs of scenes which were either the right way up or inverted and then later asked them to indicate (a) whether certain scenes had been seen before and (b) whether they had been inverted or not. The manipulation of inversion can be equated with circumstances of encounter. It was shown that while scenes were well recognized the circumstances of their encounter were not. Brown, Deffenbacher and Sturgill (1977) presented their subjects with twenty-five pictures of faces in one room and twenty-five different faces in a different room. All subjects were told to expect a later recognition test. Two days later subjects were asked (a) to say whether one of a pair of faces had been presented before and (b) in which room. Only 58 per cent correct matching of face with room of presentation was obtained, whereas 96 per cent correct recognition of faces previously seen was achieved. Now this theory, as a demonstrable fact, suggests that poor memory ought to be the rule rather than the exception in real-life situations because rarely is the situation of identification the same as the situation of viewing. Further, while the viewing of crimes is of a dynamic event and person, the situation of identification is either a static mugshot or a static parade. Both of these, on the encoding specificity hypothesis account, would produce poor memory.

Motivated forgetting

A complete account of remembering and forgetting cannot ignore what the person is trying to do – both when he remembers and when he forgets. The notion of repression suggests that some memories become inaccessible because of the way they relate to our personal feelings. Memories can be forgotten because they are unacceptably associated with guilt and anxiety. Now while repression is at base a Freudian concept and thus problematic for hard-nosed experimentalists its existence has been validated by, among others, Kline (1972). Clinical evidence also exists for its reality and the amnesic syndrome is good evidence. Amnesia can stem from physical trauma such as a blow on the head, or a fall, but occassionally one finds amnesia brought on by great emotional shock. In these cases forgetting is highly selective and focused – the memories forgotten being those referring to the self – one's name, family, home address, personal biography. Psychotherapy is full of such cases. This type of memory disruption can also be related to criminal cases and the nature and amount of testimony of witnesses. Kuehn (1974) showed that women are poorer than men at describing their assailants and this cannot be explained either by the type of crime or the nature of the injury. It could be that women to a large extent repress memories and perceptions associated with an emotional situation more than men. Other explanations are of course possible and we will look at these more carefully later in this chapter, and Chapter 7.

All these theories of forgetting have some validity but no one theory explains all the facts of eyewitness testimony in all cases. All the theories have application to person identification. The greater the time between initial perception of a criminal and eventual identification the greater the danger will be of faulty memory. The greater the similiarity of intervening events and people between perception and recognition the greater is the chance of distortion and forgetting due to interference. Systematic distortion of the memory trace is a well exhibited fact and its understanding is clearly of importance to the defence and prosecution. Similarly retrieval failure is a real-life problem. The Tip of the Tongue (TOT) phenomena elucidated by Brown and McNeill (1964) is an experience we have all had and the methods people go through to extricate themselves from this unpleasant state are instructive. They use many cues which appear to be unrelated to the immediate task. As an example of this Yarmey (1973) used famous faces and showed that linguistic, phonological, situational and occupational cues were all associated with a stored visual trace of a face which at a particular moment in time was inaccessible. These findings suggest that the belief that faces are stored solely in some visual form is unacceptable. One most instructive phenomenological observation with the TOT phenomena is that a solution is usually achieved by turning away from an attempted recall, 'forget about it for a second and it will come' is a frequent statement by a person in the situation. This suggests that a focusing of attention which is usually necessary for adequate retrieval may, in fact, be counterproductive in certain situations. The implication of this is that perhaps a relaxed, leisurely atmosphere in police stations with the absence of uniforms and official paraphernalia may be a conducive atmosphere for adequate person or event identification or recollection. In this relaxed atmosphere potential recall or recognition cues would have a greater effect. Perhaps hypnosis produces such benefits because it operates in precisely these relaxed situations. Motivated forgetting again is a real problem for the police because if repression operates immediately after a traumatic or emotional event the witness may produce such statements as 'I cannot remember a thing' but if later, when the shock has worn off, he can produce a fairly good description of people and events, a defence counsel could with great effect argue that the witness's later testimony was in fact nothing but confabulation, whereas an awareness of the emotional basis of memory would suggest that, while it could be confabulation, it could also be the result of subsiding emotion and ego defence with the concomitant rising to awareness of the perceived, encoded and stored events which produced the initial emotion.

A cautionary note on method and theory

Now it has often been said that while these theories of forgetting are useful general frameworks within which to view the possible sources of eyewitness unreliability, the more specific research endeavours of experimental psychologists have been less than helpful. This was essentially the position taken by Devlin (1976). This stems from a number of sources, chief amongst which is the mode of carrying on academic research which tends to be theory-testing orientated, based on a consideration of formal elegance, logical rigour and intersubjective verification, thus tending to dispense with problem-centred studies which are concerned to be situationally valid, socially relevant and productive of publicly usable knowledge. Thus, much of the research in memory, although ingeniously planned and painstakingly executed, could be argued to have little relevance for eyewitness testimony. Pure research, while at base a necessary condition for fruitful applied research, suffers from the restriction of the number of independent variables employed in the laboratory; from too severe control over variables, which eventuate in findings of no practical importance; from the choosing of the dependent variable in terms of convenience rather than importance, and the presentation of stimuli of an artifical nature in an unrealistic way. While we do not subscribe to this view in its entirety there is more than a grain of truth in it. Early psychological studies of memory were concerned to answer the question how and why we forget. They produced some possible accounts, which we have reviewed briefly above, but then instead of looking at these in terms of generality and generalizability, experimental psychologists began to focus on the way these theories of forgetting explained the types of experiments they were conducting. Broadly speaking, experimental psychologists have presented groups of stimuli for very short exposure durations (less than a second) and then asked for immediate recall of all or part of the presented stimuli. Another research paradigm developed wherein items were presented one by one in list form and then recall of these items was asked for within a short time (0–30 seconds). A third approach to the study of memory has been to have subjects learn, to some criterion, a set of stimuli and then test for memory at some more or less later date (one minute to 3–4 weeks). These techniques became associated with memory structures referred to respectively as sensory stores which held material only briefly, short-term stores which held material for medium lengths of time (0–30 seconds), if not rehearsed or repeated, and long-term stores which held material for long periods of time, being based on organizational processes. A huge number of experimental man-hours became invested in this Paradigm-Structure-Characteristics circuit. The problem is that it seemed to have very little relevance to the psychology of person identification in particular and eyewitness memory in general. It was felt that this research effort left the potentially rich reciprocity between experimental psychology and law enforcement extremely sterile. Over and above the 'locking in' on limited paradigms and discrete boxes (stores) the prevailing custom was to use verbal material. Because person identification was essentially visual any research which dealt with verbal material must be irrelevant. It will be argued theoretically and shown experimentally that this divide and conquer attitude is wrong and it can be shown logically that, at the very least, the verbal and visual memory systems interact, because we can talk about seen events and we can imagine scenes which we read about. Because research was not directly applied and based on a 'problem approach', an overgeneralized view was that experimental psychology was in danger of becoming lost in theoretical obscurity, failing to see the important applied forest for unimportant or trivial laboratory trees. This we do not accept. A great deal of the knowledge gained from pure memory research on verbal material predicts, at least qualitatively, many of the findings which have emerged from both pure research with visual material, and more applied research with real-life events and people. What will be shown to differ is the precise qualification of man's memory ability under different conditions.

To reject the great wealth of information contained within academic psychology would be a grave mistake because even while becoming 'too narrow' in interest and focus this research effort held the seeds of its own recovery. Scientific progress is always based on a huge edifice of error: psychology has now realized that it may have been wrong in its stress on structure. Craik and Lockhart (1972) proposed a new framework within which to view memory and memory research. The method of future progress was argued to be a concentration on process rather than structure; boxes with their own characteristics were seen as a theoretical dead-end. The person in any encounter with reality tries to abstract the meaning or essence of what is happening or has happened. It is this meaning or essence, together with the more or less accurate memory of the actual details which implied that meaning, which is stored. If it can be accepted that memory is concerned with storing meaning then it should matter little whether the actual form of the input is visual or verbal. Much the same theoretical position has been arrived at by Restle (1974) who talks of 'degrees of organization' by which he means that the memorizer is concerned to relate progressively the input to his already available existing experience. Man's existing stock of knowledge is used to direct perception, encode events and assimilate experience.

Thus it is now realized that man perceives and conceives the new through the old. This is a crucial insight for the psychology of person recognition. All that remains to be achieved now is for psychologists to accept that they cannot divide thinking, perceiving and memorizing man from feeling, believing, striving man. Chapter 3 will make this clear but for the moment let us see just what psychological studies have to say about how good visual memory is, what are its important determinants and whether laboratory man is the same creature as real-life man in his memory for faces and events.

Memory for visual input: persons and events

Laboratory studies

While there has been a massive growth in memory research it is fairly true to say (as we have indicated above) that the majority of such research has been conducted with verbal material and thus could be called irrelevant. But if, as we argued earlier, the memory system has a common function, the abstraction and storage of meaning, then it should matter little what form the input takes and thus the laws of verbal memory should predict the findings in visual memory, at least qualitatively.

Where visual material has been used memory has been shown to be extremely good – at least in the laboratory, but as we will show later this is a very important caveat. The basic procedure used to test visual memory is to present subjects with a large number of pictures of various scenes, objects and faces and then at some later time to ask them to indicate those seen pictures from a group of previously seen pictures and previously unseen pictures. One researcher, Shepard (1967), asked people to look at 600 pictures of various objects, landscapes and scenes. They were then shown 60 pairs of pictures where only one of each member of a pair had been seen in the original 600. They were simply asked, for each pair, to pick out the previously seen picture. This situation is quite analagous to going through a series of mugshots. Correct identification was made in 97 per cent of the cases. In a similar type of experiment Nickerson (1965) showed 800 pictures of objects to a group of people and then showed them another set of 400 pictures and they had to say which of these 400 pictures had appeared in the first batch of seen photos. For the second part of the experiment he varied the number of intervening pictures before the initially seen pictures reappeared. (This is a manipulation which systematically varies the time between initial viewing and later identification and is closely analogous to identification parades carried out at varying lengths of time since the initial perception of the criminal.) Nickerson noted 97 per cent correct identification with a lag of 40 pictures and 87 per cent correct identification with a lag of 200. Thus, as work on verbal memory would suggest, delay since seeing the picture produces a decrement in memory, but note that this decrease in performance is not large, and in fact it could be argued that delay has no effect. Seeking the limits of visual memory, Standing, Conezio and Haber (1970) showed to a group of students the staggering total of 2,500 photos of unfamiliar paintings, scenes and magazine photos each for 5–10 seconds. At the end of about seven hours' viewing the observers still achieved 90 per cent correct identification of seen photos, even with an interval of a day and a half between first seeing and later identifying. Increasing the number of pictures to 10,000 Standing in 1973 found accurate recognition and recall decreased to only 86 per cent correct identification. This is truly phenomenal visual memory.

Laboratory studies – faces

Only a brief summary of face research will be discussed here as a much fuller coverage is given in Chapter 4. While the power of visual memory seems staggering it could be objected that it is quite easy to distinguish between different objects – a cat is vastly different from an aeroplane. Face recognition may be quite a different story because the pattern of features are very similar across all faces. What are the facts? Hochberg and Galper (1967) asked people to look first at a series of 35 and then at a series of 60 faces. They then presented 15 pairs of photographs – one of each pair having been seen previously, the other not – and asked for identification of the previously seen face. The subjects' recognition performance was better with 35 faces than with 60 faces, but even with 60 faces to store they still recognized them on 90 per cent of occasions. In this study faces were of females. Yin (1969) observed 96 per cent correct identification of male faces presented as photographs.

Once psychologists have established the basic facts they then progress to look at factors which can either enhance or decrease performance. One such factor has already been alluded to – delay since first viewing. Laughery and his colleagues (Laughery, Alexander and Lane, 1971) have made the most systematic attack on the psychological mechanisms underlying the forgetting of faces. They looked at ability to recognize a target person from 150 pictures of faces. Again the analogy with looking through a series of mugshots should be emphasized.

They found that the longer the time for which the target person had been viewed the better was the eventual identification. They also found that the earlier the target person turned up in the identification sequence (i.e. the shorter the delay or lag) the more likely was he to be recognized. (An interesting finding was that it made no difference whether the pictures were frontal, profile or portrait.) In these studies, however, delay and interference through similarity were confounded. In 1974 Laughery tried to clarify the evidence by varying systematically the time lag between seeing a face and trying to recognize it again, and also the similarity between the target face (already seen) and the decoy faces (faces not previously seen). Delay between seeing the face and recognizing it made no difference *unless* there was a substantial similarity between the target person and the decoys. When this was the case delay did become important and damaging (Laughery, Fessler, Lenorovitz and Yoblick, 1974). This seems good evidence for the interference effect theory of forgetting outlined above, and in an unpublished PhD thesis Forbes at Aberdeen University provides some suggestive evidence for at least pro-active interference with faces.

Thus in terms of making predictions about visual memory for events and faces, verbal memory findings have been quite useful, at least qualitatively. Research with words has indicated that delay between learning and recalling is important, that substantial similarity has an interfering effect and that the larger the initial learning set the poorer the relative recall. These verbal memory predictions have been upheld in the visual studies quoted above by Shepard, Nickerson, Laughery *et al.*, and further, Yarmey (1974) found that the more recognition trials an observer undertakes the poorer becomes performance.

Visual and verbal memory – the same or different?

There is a great dearth of applied memory research in problems of person recognition, but there is a great deal of highly sophisticated 'pure research' which we argue is relevant and transferable to, but not directly derived from, such areas. To make this argument we will have to show that: (a) the belief that verbal and visual memory are different processes in essence is not tenable, and (b) that the belief that memory for visual stimuli in general is different from memory for faces is also untenable. A conception of memory will be advanced which focuses on 'meaning' with the actual form of input, verbal or visual, facial or non-facial configurations, as secondary and derivative. Before this way of conceptualizing memory can be justified and specified let us first of all briefly review the evidence which has been taken to suggest that visual and verbal storage, and also facial and non-facial storage are different and separate memory systems.

Verbal and pictorial memory

Recently, Salthouse (1974) presented evidence that, 'Verbal and pictorial information are stored and processed in separate information processing systems' and that they 'are fundamentally different in their types of memory representation'. He notes that, 'Almost all present memory theories are based entirely on research with verbal stimulus material', and because he believes that, 'Non-verbal stimuli are retained in a visual mode', he suggests that in the light of his findings present day theories of memory and information processing are in need of revision. There is certainly a substantial amount of evidence that whereas the memorability of verbal material appears to decrease with time between initial presentation and the later recognition test, that for pictorial stimuli may not. Laughery *et al.* (1974) found no effect of delays (of 4 minutes, 30 minutes, 1 hour, 4 hours, 1 day, 1 week) upon facial recognition performance but they note that many experiments employing verbal material have observed effects of delays. Shepherd and Ellis (1973) found no overall effect of delay across an interval of one month, and Goldstein and Chance (1971) found no effect of a 48-hour delay. The latter authors concluded that, 'these data suggest that pictorial stimuli may not need the assistance of verbal material for storage and retrieval from memory.' Scapinello and Yarmey (1970) and Yarmey (1971) observed no effect of delays of 20 minutes which led Yarmey to state that, 'These data partially support Goldstein and Chance (1971) who found that verbal mediation did not improve recognition memory for pictorial stimuli.' In another study Yarmey (1973) again stated that, 'In the last ten years other memory systems, particularly nonverbal imagery, have been rediscovered and shown to be equally important in memory tasks.' In his particular study portrait photographs of famous persons were presented and the subjects were asked to try to put a name to the face. However, his own evidence strongly implicates verbal coding in visual memory. He believes that, 'other information such as phonemic information is often available', and in fact concludes that, 'Subjects descriptions of their memory search during "tip of the tongue" states clearly involved both imagery and verbal mediators.'

Thus many authors now believe that there exists a pictorial memory, and this process seems exceedingly efficient at recognizing faces. However, as Goldstein and Chance (1974) point out (having modified their views of 1971), the notion of there being two separate memory systems, verbal vs. pictorial, is almost exclusively based on the apparent superior performance of the latter and its remaining untouched by the passage of time. These authors now believe that the observed differences in performances are artifactual and are a function of: (i) the need in verbal recognition tests to be able to remember almost the whole stimuli (because many of the 100,000 words in the English language are very alike) whereas with pictures, which are more variable, fewer aspects of the total stimulus are usually required for correct recognition; (ii) in the delay studies, during the interval between initial presentation and test, there is more chance of the subjects' encountering stimuli similar to the presented verbal material than stimuli similar to the verbal material and consequently interference will be greater in the former. Thus Goldstein and Chance now believe that there is in fact no evidence for the existence of two different sorts of memory.

From the practical point of view it is very important to be able to decide whether there exists a purely pictorial memory process. Present police methods of gathering descriptive information frequently involve asking witnesses for verbal descriptions. One of the major problems in this area is determining to what extent pictorial input and output can be the result of a translation to and from a verbal mode (the verbal-loop hypothesis of Glanzer and Clark, 1964). If such translation occurs it seems almost impossible to observe it experimentally. It is probable that some occurs but its extent is as yet unknown. Frijda and Van de Geer (1961) believe that visual recognition of facial expression can be a function of verbal codability but they offer no evidence of the extent to which this occurs and the stages (input, storage, retrieval) at which it operates. Nielsen and Smith (1973) claim that for short delays (ten seconds) the memory of a face is likely to be purely visual. They found visual recognition reaction times to be independent of the number of factors causing the variance in the array of faces in the recognition test, and that reaction times and errors when recognizing drawings of faces were less if the initial presentation were a photograph of the face than if it were a verbal description of the face. Such findings present problems for those who claim that we translate from visual input to verbal coding. Howells (1938) also found evidence that there may be two separate memory systems since he noted that, 'Subjects who were superior in naming details of facial photographs were not superior at recognition.' Also Malpass, Lavigueur and Weldon (1973) found that training in giving verbal descriptions of faces did not improve visual recognition performance. Thus even when verbal labels for pictorial input were provided performance did not improve.

It seems probable that we can remember things that are in fact difficult to put into words. Later (Chapter 4) we shall examine whether faces are remembered by single features or by the patterning between features but it is worth stating now that it is a well-documented psychological finding that patterns and configurations are extremely difficult to represent in words (Liggett, 1974). As Bourne (1966) suggests, sometimes, 'verbal labels do not exist because the stimulus attributes do not lend themselves easily to verbal associations.' Roger Brown, along with others, has suggested that the length of response (assessed in several ways), is an index of the codability of stimuli. The shorter the response the more codable the stimulus, and presumably the higher its availability to the subject. Chance and Goldstein (1976) asked subjects to label faces and they found that the labels were compounds (more than one word) on 65 per cent of occasions when the label had to describe the face, and 85 per cent when their subjects had to say what the face reminded them of. This suggests that verbal codes for faces are not readily available to most subjects, a compound set of words being a weaker coding than a single word. Upon request most people say that they can in fact conjure up in their mind's eye a truly visual image of someone they know though usually this image fades very quickly. If such a phenomenon really exists, its harnessing could be of great value. Salthouse (1974) believes that most people do experience truly visual images and Haber (1969) claims eidetic imagery is a real phenomenon (although we will have occasion to question this in Chapter 7). He notes that, 'the eidetic child pays no attention to his eidetic image when organizing his verbal memory', and that, 'the shunning by psychologists of such an interesting topic as eidetic imagery should be ended'. Even though only a small percentage of the population may possess full-blown eidetic powers it might be worth while to place these persons in occupations where such talents can be usefully employed.

Now it can be said that the above studies are compatible with the argument for separate processing accounts of visual and verbal material but they do not prove that there are in fact two distinct types of processing involved. The difference between visual and verbal memory may be only a difference of degree not of kind and in support of this it ought to be pointed out that Goldstein and Chance (1971) give clear evidence of very poor picture memory and Jenkins, Stack and Deno (1969) showed that the memory performance of 7-year-old children was no better for pictures than for words, and Ducharme and Fraisse (1965) likewise found no difference in recall of pictures and name stimuli among children aged 8 to 10 years.

It does not seem necessary to argue for separate processing systems and indeed the chief proponent of dual processing modes, Paivio (1969, 1971, 1976), bases his whole theory on the imageability of concrete *words*. He argues that the superiority of visual memory over verbal memory is due to double encoding (i.e. the storing of a scene, event or picture in both a visual and a verbal form). Various forms of the double encoding hypothesis have been suggested by a variety of authors, e.g. Sampson (1970), Bower (1972) and Wallach and Averbach (1955). The basic argument is that pictures of familiar objects or the objects themselves can be readily coded and stored in memory in a verbal form and, in addition, these objects or their pictures associatively arouse concrete images of the thing they represent. Recall or recognition probability is then higher because the memory can be retrieved from either symbolic mode (the visual or the verbal). We might ask what evidence exists for this dual encoding hypothesis. There is a lot of inference but little hard experimental evidence, and, in fact, there is some evidence that (a) it does not occur at all, or (b) if it does occur it is mediated by other factors. The evidence that it does not occur on all occasions when it should, according to Paivio, comes from the work of Nelson and his co-workers (Nelson and Brooks, 1973; Nelson and Reed, 1976). They were able to show, using techniques which need not be gone into here, that pictures of common objects apparently function as effective memory representations without evoking their corresponding name codes. This study thus suggests separate visual and verbal memory stores. The evidence that dual coding even if it does occur is not the whole story comes from Davies, Milne and Glennie (1973) who compared memory for (i) pictures alone, (ii) pictures plus their descriptive label, (iii) descriptive labels plus their referents (photos) and (iv) name alone. The dual encoding hypothesis would predict that (ii) and (iii) should not differ – both produce dual encoding. However, Davies *et al.* argued that when encoding pictures adults go beyond the evidence given to actively retrieve and generate the appropriate name. It is the active generation rather than the production of the name as such which is crucial. This view would predict that (ii) should be better than (iii) and this is precisely what was found. Thus double encoding by itself does not ensure effective recall and recognition, rather the subject must actively generate the verbal label himself. This stress on the importance of the subject actively responding to the perceptual situation has been argued by, among others, Bruner (1961, 1974) and Gropper (1963), and once again this would have been predicted from research in verbal memory where Bobrow and Bower (1969) noted better recall of a pair of nouns when subjects generated their own linking sentence than when they were given an equally appropriate one from the experimenter. Thus, while dual coding (the best currently accepted explanation of the superiority of visual memory) may go on, it is the active nature of the encoding which is necessary, at least with pictures of objects. While active processing may be a necessary condition of good picture memory, is it sufficient? And further, does this active processing also apply to face recognition? It seems that it does. Bower and Karlin (1974) presented pictures of faces to two groups of subjects, one group simply being instructed to label the picture male or female, the other group being instructed to label the faces for likeableness or honesty. The argument here is that judgments of 'what sex' require less deep processing than judgments of honesty and likeability. If Craik and Lockhart (1972) are correct there ought to be more permanent memory traces for the deeper processing group. This is what was found. Recognition accuracy was greater for those faces rated for honesty rather than sex. Thus while both groups of subjects actively encoded, it seems that 'actively' in its turn must be further broken down. Other studies have also shown that it is not merely the presence of labels but the actual type of label generated which is crucial. Chance and Goldstein (1976) showed that instructing subjects to 'write some one thing about the face which you believe will help you recognize it when you see it again' produced better recognition than merely telling subjects to either judge the ages of faces, or to write 'some one thing which the face reminds you of or looks like to you'. Other studies of face labelling will be discussed in Chapter 4.

Thus, from these studies two important factors emerge: an active subject, and an active subject who processes material to a deeper level. The question that can then legitimately be asked is, what is this 'deeper level'? It is argued that the dispute over two codes or one is something of a red herring in the search for understanding of real-life memory. Perhaps the predilection to dichotomize has hidden the fact that there is but one code which incorporates both visual and verbal parameters and perhaps the deeper encoding or storage format is abstract and conceptual, concerned with meaning. Experimental facts and logical inferences do not rule out this possibility and in fact they suggest that it is perhaps valid. Clark and Chase (1972) and Pylyshyn (1973), amongst others, have argued that conversion from one code to the other is achieved via mediation by a common abstract system in which meaning of words, sentences and pictures are represented in a modality free propositional format. If this is the case then perception ought to be facilitated by the existing schemata or the models we have in our head and with which we interpret the world (e.g. Gregory, 1974). Schemata refer to internal structures developed through experience with the world which organize incoming information relative to previous experiences. One obvious prediction from this theory is that recognition memory for organized scenes ought to be better than for disorganized scenes. If there is a visual memory and no deeper, more conceptual, propositional storage format, then no differences in recall or recognition should exist between organized and disorganized scenes because the visual details are similar in both cases, what differs is the unity of the two scenes. Mandler and Stein (1974) and Mandler and Parker (1976) put these alternative predictions to the test. They presented subjects with organized and disorganized photographs and tested for recognition of changes of their constituent elements. They found that changes in organized scenes were better recognized when they involved spatial locations but changes were much more difficult to detect when they were changes in size, shape, etc. The argument being advanced here is that where existing schemata operate they do so to maximize perception, storage and recall; where schemata are not present memory will be poor. Schemata exist for spatial arrangements especially top, bottom, horizontal, vertical and so on but schemata for sizes, except in the crudest form, do not exist and therefore memory for actual size is poor. Another group of studies which drive the same conclusion comes from Biederman (1972; Biederman, Glass and Stacy, 1973). In these studies it was demonstrated that object identification was facilitated when the objects were embedded in coherent real-world scenes compared to jumbled versions of the same scenes. It was concluded that the contextual information provided by the coherent scenes facilitated the perceptual identification of the target objects, by evoking pre-existing schemata. More directly related to person identification is the case in eyewitness testimony of recall of the criminal's size, weight and height. What one finds is that eyewitnesses report known population norms when they are unsure but being pressed to say something. The inferential reasoning which seems to go on in a witness's head is that if he cannot recall a particular attribute (e.g. height or weight), then it must be that this attribute was not outstanding or abnormal. If not abnormal what is normal? By reference to existing schemata one gets average heights and so the witness outputs these schemata-generated (supposed perceptual) memories. This is a clear case of 'perception' of the new through the old which we elaborated on above. Dunaway (1973) is one of the very few researchers to have looked at the relationship between the accuracy of height estimation as a function of several variables, among which were sex of the observer, height of the observer, and height and weight of the person being estimated. Both males and females underestimated the height of the taller targets and both sexes overestimated the height of the shorter targets. The errors made by short observers were of the same type but were more extreme, i.e. the short persons underestimated the height of a tall target more than did the taller observers. Another example, this time as applied to identification parades, can be drawn from the study by Doob and Kirshenbaum (1973) who investigated the situation in which a criminal witness had encoded a face in terms of a word which in turn represented a conceptual meaning, proposition or description, the word being 'good-looking' (this being all she could remember about the robber). The shop girl, when asked to attend a police identification parade, picked out a person who was rated by forty-one non-involved students at a later date as the best looking. Doob and Kirshenbaum argued that this could be due to a schema, labelled 'good looking', being the only stored representation that the witness had of the criminal and thus being matched to a line-up with persons of differential facial attractiveness. The true criminal need not have been present to have someone picked out. This study will be more closely examined in Chapter 6.

The psychology of visual memory is further advanced by borrowing from an area of study which has had a great influence on the study of verbal memory. This is the area of psycholinguistics and the borrowed concepts are 'surface structure' and 'deep structure' as proposed by Chomsky (1957, 1965). The surface structure of a sentence is the form and wording of a sentence. Thus an active sentence would be 'The boy kicked the ball' and a passive sentence would be 'The ball was kicked by the boy'. While the surface structure of the two sentences differ (active or passive), the meaning (factual content) in terms of actions and actors is basically the same. However, do note that we are not at all well informed about characteristics of either the boy, the ball or the type of kick. It could be this intrinsically greater potential for certainty (Clifford and Collier, in preparation) which a picture contains, as compared to a sentence, that accounts for the exhibited superiority of visual memory over verbal memory. This seems a fruitful hypothesis because the number of inferences and implications that can be drawn from a sentence is quite large. Consider the different inferences and images that one conjures up when the two following sentences are read:

The king was eating his dinner
The baby was eating his dinner

The potential inferences concerning the 'mess', 'splendour' and type of food being eaten would be greatly reduced if pictures of the two diners were presented. We would be more certain of what was the case and thus our stored memories would be clearer.

This distinction between surface structure and deep structure is not too radical because it has been argued that the human being has evolved to deal with symbols, and symbols are concerned with meaning, form being secondary – we stop at traffic lights, at verbal stop signs and at the raised hand of a policeman. As shown above it makes little difference to understanding whether we hear an active or a passive sentence, and in studies of verbal memory surface form is quickly lost (Sachs, 1967, 1974; Wanner, 1974) whereas meaning is retained. Baggett (1975) in a nice experiment shows clearly the possibility of separating out (i) a sensory representation of individual pictures of events, (ii) a conceptual representation of the individual pictures, and (iii) the explicit and implicit inferences contained in the series formed by these individual pictures when they are grouped into a series to tell a story. Both Baggett (1975) and Nelson and Reed (1976) suggest that visual superiority may reside in the sensory attributes of the perceived stimulus because they are more differentiating than those of a corresponding label describing these events. However, at long lags between initial perception and later recognition it is the conceptual, propositional, level which is crucial, and it is long delays between seeing a criminal act and recognizing the criminal which is the rule rather than the exception in real life. (The Devlin Report suggests an average of four weeks.) But not only the delay is crucial, surface structure will become relatively less important and the conceptual level more important when the stimuli are rather similar (such as faces), or the perception is fleeting (such as eyewitness perception of criminal episodes) and thus the meaning which the viewer imparts to the situation, and his total cognitive system, become crucial determinants of accuracy and reliability of person identification. That surface structure features of pictures of faces are not too crucial was shown by Harmon (1973) who noted that people immediately recognized uniformally degraded, blurred photographs of Lincoln and the Mona Lisa, where no surface structure features existed. The usual glib explanation of this finding is that they are very familiar photographs – but how familiar is familiar? Have you seen photographs of either of these two people more than five times? It seems that there is something else stored about these people which aids rapid recognition – it cannot be surface structure features. Is it mood, bearing, meaning?

Visual and face memory – the same or different?

The thesis developed above, whereby memory was argued to be an abstractive constructive process based on meaning, was seen to be valid in terms of verbal memory, and if it is accepted that verbal and visual memory do not differ except perhaps quantitively, then by extrapolation it is applicable to visual memory also. In order to extrapolate even further there remains one hurdle to jump – the possibility that face memory is somehow qualitatively different from visual memory *per se*. This question has been most adequately reviewed by Ellis (1975) upon whom this account draws.

There is a substantial amount of research which suggests that facial memory is mediated by processes which are different from the processes that underlie visual memory in general. One such difference is suggested by Bradshaw and Wallace (1971) who asked subjects to rapidly compare pairs of identikit faces, that varied on a number of possible different features from two to seven, and to say whether the faces in each pair were the same or different. From their data Bradshaw and Wallace concluded that recognition of faces involves very fast processing, employing serial search rather than parallel search of the different features within a face. The focus of this section will be on whether it is possible to reject the idea that faces are a unique pattern of features which are processed by a uniquely developed mechanism involving face-specific analysers. As Ellis (1975) points out the belief that there are unique face-specific analysers is derived from three principal sources: (i) the ontogeny of facial recognition, (ii) experiments involving inversion of faces and (iii) clinical evidence from prosopagnosia, a psychology defect which is characterized by an inability to recognize the most familiar of faces.

Ontogeny Bond (1972) surveyed the vast literature which exists to show that infants respond to faces at a very early age, but he also made clear that while the facts are evident the explanation is problematical. Carpenter (1974; Carpenter, Tecce, Stechler and Friedman, 1970) indicates that within the first two weeks babies are able to differentiate their mother's face from a model of a face and a non-facial model. Wolff (1963) indicated that within four weeks babies smile in response to a face, and Fantz's (e.g. 1961) extensive work has clearly shown that babies respond to 'face like' stimuli preferentially. The great problem in this type of research, as pointed out by Salapatek and Kesson (1966), and reaffirmed by Bond (1972), is that we may be building in too grandiose anthropomorphic assumptions as to just what the baby is doing. It may simply be the case that babies are responding to some general difference among classes of stimuli, such as brightness or transitional zones, rather than to the pattern detail. The difficulty of using ontogenetic explanations is that they are very hard to falsify due to the difficulty of creating an appropriately controlled experiment. Once again the black or white approach – learned or innate – hides many shades of grey. These shades of grey have been spelt out by Blakemore (1973) and provide rather clear guidelines for adequate research, but ethical considerations constrain human research. Where ethics are involved psychologists traditionally retreat to animal studies hoping that extrapolative interest will hide the problem of dubiety stemming from the fact that even intra-species differences are very marked. To achieve useful data we must continue to experiment with human neonates. The answer lies in tighter methodology such as that by Haaf (1974; Haaf and Brown, 1976), who shows clearly that length of fixation is related to stimulus complexity but not to the degree of facial resemblance of stimuli in neonates of five to ten weeks.

Thus the evidence for an innate basis to face perception is fraught with difficulties. Baby research and methodological problems always allow of alternative interpretation, and phylogenetic extrapolation is at best doubtful.

Inversion of faces It is generally the case that visual perception is reasonably good for both upright and inverted stimuli – note how easily you can read this book upside down. One class of stimuli not so equally recognized is faces (Goldstein, 1965; Hochberg and Galper, 1967). This specific (face) deficit has been ascribed to the operation of face-specific analysers.

Theorists who want to postulate specific face analysers are, however, at odds with one another. Yin (1969, 1970) and Konorski (1967) both postulate innate analysers for faces – but whilst Konorski predicts that inverted facial recognition should be better than recognition of inverted pictures of objects usually found in one plane only (e.g. trees and buildings), Yin found quite the opposite to be the case. Konorski is arguing that the specific face analysers are more flexible than the analysers which are 'switched in' for familiar objects; Yin is arguing, at least implicitly, quite the opposite.

A group of studies relevant to this whole area of research is the work of Stratton (1897) with inverting spectacles and the related studies of Kohler (1962). It was found that the initial wearing of prismatic spectacles greatly disorientated the wearer – but, and this is the important point, the disorientation was soon overcome. Thus visual analysers dealing with visual objects which normally had a fixed orientation could be re-educated. Can face analysers also be re-educated? It seems as if they can. Bradshaw and Wallace (1971) showed that with practice their subjects could greatly improve their rate of searching inverted faces. Thus both general visual and specific facial analysers, if such a distinction exists, can be re-educated. The possibility of re-education casts doubt on the innate basis of special facial analysers. Thus the findings of Yin (1969) and Scapinello and Yarmey (1970) can be explained by learned habits of perceiving faces, and other visual objects, plus the greater complexity of faces compared with other visual objects. Rock (1974) indicates

47

that mental rotation of any figure with multiple components would be harder than a figure with few components, and this seems to account for the difficulty experienced with faces.

Children are frequently a non-confirmatory test-bed for research and theory carried out on adults. However, even here research is conflicting. Brooks and Goldstein (1963) showed a positive relationship to exist between age of observer and recognition of inverted classmates' faces, while Goldstein (1965) showed that children are less inhibited by inverted faces than are adults. The latter result is predicated upon, and predicted from, an argument in terms of 'opportunity for learning' and as such is neutral on the question of innate and/or specific facial analysers. The explanation of the difference between the two studies could be one of familiarity. The older you are the longer you have been with classmates and therefore the more familiar you are with classmates' faces, in all types of orientation. Thus, like the ontogenetic argument, the inverted face research fails to provide unequivocal evidence for a unique, perhaps innate set of facial analysers.

Prosopagnosia Prosopagnosia is a clinically recognized condition characterized by an inability to recognize faces of familiar acquaintances. Because of the nature of the condition some researchers have been led to postulate the existence of face-specific analysers which are either destroyed or damaged in patients exhibiting the symptoms of prosopagnosia (Hecaen and Angelergues, 1962; Konorski, 1967; Yin, 1970). The simplicity of this idea is appealing but not without its problems. Functional specificity often carries the connotation of localization of function. However, the literature on prosopagnosia gives diverse anatomical locations (see Ellis, 1975 for review), and anyway the logic of 'sites' or 'centres' for brain functioning is not compelling: pathways can easily be misleadingly labelled 'sites'.

The characteristic defects in face recognition of prosopagnosia patients is both interesting and instructive. A useful heuristic tool of psychologists is to extrapolate from abnormal functioning to normal functioning, and if this is a valid form of advance then specific complaints in prosopagnosia are highly suggestive for future research and predictive of present research yet to be discussed. For example, some patients refer to great difficulty with eye regions (Gloning, Gloning, Hoff and Tschabitscher, 1966), but for others the eyes are the easiest (Hecaen and Angelergues, 1962).

The interesting thing about prosopagnostics is that they always say they cannot recognize faces. Thus at least a two-stage process of face perception must be postulated: the detection of the presence of a face and then further analysis during which information is extracted concerning various other features and finally a match is made with any stored memory trace of that particular face.

Bay (1953) argued that prosopagnosia may be due to a failure to integrate various parts of the face into a whole, while Faust (1947) suggested that prosopagnosia was characterized by a failure to grasp the detailed features of a complex pattern so that its uniqueness could be encoded, and reported a patient who failed not only to identify faces but to distinguish a chair from an armchair, indicating 'a more general perceptual deficit' (Ellis, 1975). It is also possible that this represents a semantic deficit, and thus it may be the meaning level that is disturbed in cases of prosopagnosia, and indeed De Renzi and Spinnler (1966) argued, due to the correlation between deficits with both face and non-face stimuli, that prosopagnosia may be a deficiency in high-level integration of visual data, and this is not face specific.

Thus the conclusion to be drawn in terms of the question as to whether visual memory and face memory are mediated by the same or different processes is that the evidence for unique face analysers is at best not strong and highly equivocal. Thus Ellis (1975) concludes that there is no good reason for supposing that the recognition and storage of faces basically differs from that involved when other visual information is presented. Indeed the ability of faces to interfere retro-actively with the memory of geometric patterns as shown by Cohen and Granstrom (1970) suggests some communality of processing for both types of material. Ellis states, 'The upshot of this conclusion is that facial recognition is likely to be subject to similar independent variables as those affecting the recognition of other complex visual stimuli', and we would add that the interpretation of the dependent variable will be similar to that found in visual memory in general, and in verbal memory.

REAL-LIFE MEMORY

So far then we have looked at the experimental evidence which shows that visual memory is very good, and that face memory reflects this general ability of humans. If these laboratory findings can be validated then identification parades, photo-fit construction, mugshot recognition, and furnishing of descriptions to the police of seen criminals should be a formality and justice should be carried out with no inherent danger. The problem is that the laboratory levels of performance are not observed in real-life settings.

In this area of investigation there are many differences between laboratory experiments and real-life situations, but four are of signal importance. In the laboratory situation inspection time is greatly extended as compared to that of the real-life incident where the face comes out of the blue and disappears with the same suddenness. The second main difference lies in the total 'atmosphere'. Laboratories are not emotionally charged but crime episodes are, and the eyewitness is left with an aftermath of outrage, confusion, fear and shock. Third, no threat is being implied in the laboratory whereas in real life often the key witness was the centre of emotional trauma by virtue of being the victim. The last obvious difference between the laboratory and reality is that in real-life incidents the victim or bystander perceives a 'face-in-motion' but is then asked to recognize or recall a static face or photograph. Usually in laboratory studies the 'stimulus' and the 'response' photo is one and the same and they are static.

The above four differences are rather easy to discern but more subtle differences also exist which are linked to the above points. The perceiver in the non-stressful laboratory will be using maximally efficient cognitive strategies to process and store the face, whereas the victim or the naive bystander will be undergoing diffuse anxiety reactions which are not conducive to maximally efficient strategies of memorization. This highlighting of the *emotional* context of a basically rational cognitive act of perceiving, storing and remembering indicates where present psychological research into face perception has been misled. Mostly researchers have been content to transfer wholesale the mechanisms of decay and interference, found useful in verbal memory research, into the area of visual memory, and to suggest that these are the necessary and sufficient explanations for poor witness reliability. But this will not do.

What research into witness identification needs to take account of is the total emotional atmosphere of the situation, plus the fact that a conceptual distinction must be made between the nominal stimulus (face as presented) and the functional stimulus (face as perceived by victim and bystander). Perceptual input is always perceived in terms of the person's existing cognitive structure, and this cognitive structure is flexible. Under conditions of stress, anxiety and fear the level of cognitive complexity used to perceive with may be very sub-optimal. A study which hints at this is one by Kuehn (1974) where he concludes from a survey of police records that perception of criminal assailants is dependent on several variables, one of which is the nature of the crime. Phenomenologically it seems that crimes can be ranged along a continuum of emotional loading – the more emotion-provoking crimes being the least well remembered (robberies produce better descriptions than rapes and assaults), A further interesting aspect of this study was the better memory of male victims than of female victims which cannot be ascribed to either type of crime or injury to the victim. Kuehn tentatively concludes that the poor recollection by females may be due to socialization practices wherein females learn to be more fearful, vulnerable and less capable in violent encounters. This finding should be compared with laboratory studies, which we will review presently, where, in non-stress situations, females are better than men at recognizing faces.

The prediction from this comparison between real-life and laboratory memorization is that very rapidly evidence will accumulate that man is not an error free recording device (the inference which could be drawn from laboratory studies, especially when one gets 86 per cent correct recognition/recall of 10,000 pictures!). Rather, simulated, 'real-life' studies will serve to demonstrate what Bruner and Postman (1949) showed a long time ago by means of an 'odd' pack of cards, namely that humans do not report what happened but rather what should have happened, i.e. 'They go beyond the information given'. Rorschach cards show quite clearly that subjects will quite happily, and readily, produce prefabrication, prevarication and coherence out of a chaotic ink blot. Memory comprises the original stimulus situation and inferences drawn after the fact.

The usual situation in simulated crime cases is to stage some incident (which has been carefully planned and is closely monitored) in front of a group of unsuspecting witnesses, and then at some later date either to ask for remembered details of actions or people, to present photos one of which was the criminal and ask for recognition, or to form an identification parade and ask the witnesses to pick out the criminal. This experimental approach is a big advance over static inspection and recognition of photographs in the sense that the action is dynamic, it reproduces real life in content and subjects' unpreparedness for becoming witnesses, and, because it is experimental, very careful checks can be made on all aspects of the perception, memory and identification processes especially the rating data given by witnesses as to their certainty of correctness. Because it is staged, the conceptual problem of distinguishing between perception and memory is side-stepped – one ensures that the witnesses perceive the indicent because it is protracted well beyond that of most real-life crimes. (It should be noted that this manipulation and others associated with the experimental set-up will serve to give an inflated picture of the accuracy of identification.)

Fired by the nagging gap between data on basic perceptual processes in controlled research settings and important questions about perception in the less well-controlled real-world, and inspired by the new look in perception (exemplified in the work of Neisser and Haber, Buckhout at the City University of New York embarked on a series of experiments in eyewitness testimony which should be required reading for all barristers, solicitors, judges and potential jurists. For a number of reasons his publications are not easily available in print, so a fairly full account of his quite incisive studies will be given here.

In order to study the effects of eyewitness testimony in a somewhat realistic setting Buckhout staged an assault located on the California State University campus, in which a distraught student 'attacked' a professor in front of 141 witnesses. Another outsider of the same age as the distraught student was deliberately on the scene. The whole incident was recorded on video-tape so that objective reality could be compared with the eyewitness's reports. After the attack Buckhout and his colleagues took sworn statements from each witness asking them to describe the suspect, the incident and the clothes worn. They also asked for a confidence rating of the descriptions. The witnesses gave very inaccurate descriptions, and they greatly overestimated the duration of the incident (in this case by a factor of over $2\frac{1}{2}$). The accuracy score for the appearance and dress was only 25 per cent of the maximum possible total score. Height and weight were reasonably accurate but unfortunately Buckhout had chosen a target person of average height and weight (thus there was no independent means of assessing whether subjects were perceiving and remembering accurately or merely utilizing a schemata-generated inference). Seven weeks later Buckhout presented a set of six photographs to each witness individually, creating four conditions which allowed testing of biased instruction and unfair testing of eyewitnesses (topics we will be covering later). Basically the experimenters led the witness either to expect that the suspect was in one of the photographs, or no such suggestion was made by simply asking if anyone was familiar ('biased' or 'no biased' instruction conditions). 'Leading photo' arrays had one picture (of the suspect wearing different clothes from the other persons) sitting at an angle to the other, neatly lined, photos. 'Non-leading' photo displays had all persons with the same expression, similar clothes and no misalignment. Overall, 40 per cent of the witnesses correctly identified the correct person, and 25 per cent identified the wrong man. Of the 40 per cent correct identification the highest percentage correct was under a combination of 'leading photo' and 'biased instruction'. An interesting footnote to this study was that even the professor picked out an innocent man. These biases and leading hints will be discussed more fully in Chapter 8.

In 1974 Buckhout and his co-workers had a male student appear at the door of a classroom and state that he thought he had left a book in the room during the previous class and that he would like to look for it. The instructor, who knew that the incident was staged, agreed to the request. The student then walked to a chair where a confederate of the experimenters was seated and bent over as if to look for a book. He snatched the confederate's pocketbook and fled from the room. The confederate screamed as the 'criminal' ran out of the door. The instructor cautioned the class to remain seated, and ran after the thief. A few minutes later the instructor and the experimenter returned and informed the students of the nature of the incident and distributed questionnaires. Three weeks later the experimenter again returned to the class and distributed another set of questionnaires which asked the subjects to indicate their confidence in their ability to correctly identify the 'criminal'. The subjects were then shown two videotaped line-ups and asked to pick out the 'criminal'. One line-up had the purse snatcher within it, the other line-up did not have him present. The subjects were allowed to see each line-up as many times as they needed to make a judgment (a concession to police identification parade procedures). Successful witnesses were more accurate in estimations of height and weight, and of the duration of the incident and, very suggestively, reported less stress. Successful witnesses tended to have fewer errors of omission and commission but the trend was not significant. However of the 52 witnesses, 14 selected the correct person but of these 14, 7 then went on to impeach themselves by selecting a wrong person in the blank line-up. Highly important, the 7 successful-impeached witnesses showed significantly higher confidence in their description of the criminal than the non-impeached successful witnesses. Thus overall only 13.5 per cent made an identification which was correct and not contaminated by impeachment on a later blank trial. Confidence rating here was rather poorly controlled; it consisted of simply asking the witnesses, before the line-up, how certain they were that they could pick the man out of the line-up. These ratings were compared with rating during recall and it was found that impeached witnesses had significantly higher pre-line-up confidence of recognition than during the recall, successful witnesses no difference and poor witnesses had significantly lower confidence levels per-line-up.

The line-up composition is rather important in this study but a fuller discussion will be deferred until Chapter 8 (p. 192), suffice it to say at the moment that Buckhout used five-man line-ups and in the line-up with the criminal present no look-alike was used (so providing ideal conditions for correct, high identification). Even in these conditions however only 14 out of 52 picked out the correct man, and 7 of these were untrustworthy. This is a very low percentage of person recognition.

Typically the students gave poor descriptions of suspects, show-ing a general tendency to approximate the norms for height and weight. These convenient frames of reference are the schemata to which witnesses will turn when they do not really remember precisely what the person looks like. Of great importance is the relation between confidence levels of witnesses and their actual performance. There is little support for the reliance that juries and police put on the statement, 'I'll never forget that face'. The correlations in Buckhout's data, and our own at NELP, suggest low or negative correlation between confidence in ability to recognize the criminal and the actual successful valid identi-fication of that person. Perhaps high confidence signals a witness who is only too quick to stereotype, to please the authorities or identify someone. Stylization may predispose someone to be confident but to be wrong. What could this stylization consist of? Just as cartoonists use stylization via accentuation of physical features by visual exaggeration, so witnesses may achieve stylization via application of verbal labels, or application of stereotypes. It is to the latter we now turn.

3 The influence of stereotypes on identification

In this chapter we shall attempt to illustrate the extent to which people's expectancies concerning how certain types of individuals behave can influence their perception of these individuals and their ability to recognize them. Though many studies in this area have found that observers frequently agree upon the attributes they assign to people solely on the basis of their appearance, the validity or truth of these observations often has little strength. Since art began, the role of stereotypes in predisposing observers to expect individuals to behave in certain ways has been well known, perhaps more to the actor or painter than to the audience.

One of the first psychologists to study the way in which a person's outward appearance might be related to his behaviour was Kretschmer (1936), who claimed that there was a biological reason why, for example, fat people are jolly, and tall, thin people are mean. Such ideas as these were developed further by Sheldon and Stevens (1942) who explored both the body-build categories of mesomorph (muscular), endomorph (fat) and ectomorph (thin) and the behaviours that these body builds constitutionally led people to display. Whilst Sheldon emphasized the likelihood of a biologically based relationship between appearance and behaviour he did acknowledge the possibility that society may also determine the relationship between body-build and behaviour by its expectations that people with certain appearances will behave in predictable ways (i.e. the self-fulfilling prophecy or socio-expectational model). It does seem that there is some truth in the idea of a biologically based relationship between physical appearance and behaviour and given this, the logically prior basis for society's further expectations is thus formed.

As our knowledge of the biological bases of behaviour has grown so the early idea of simple physiological relationships existing between body and behaviour has waned. However, accompanying this has been an ever strengthening belief in the socio-expectational basis for the observed relationships. Nevertheless many people are of the opinion that physical appearance and real or attributed behaviour are unrelated. This chapter will attempt to modify such views.

CRIMINALS

In 1962 Kozeny obtained photographs of 730 convicted criminals which he then divided into sixteen categories depending upon the type of crime which had been committed. From each of these sixteen groups of photographs a composite portraiture was made and these 'demonstrated statistically significant dependence of the resultant physiognomic character upon the respective category of crime from which the criminal's pictures had been taken'. Should it therefore be concluded that the people who commit crimes are of similar appearance? To some observers this might seem an unlikely state of affairs; but remember the earlier example of a mugger – are muggers all of youngish appearance? 'Modern criminologists do not believe that criminals belong to a single physical or psychological type' (Liggett, 1974), but does the general public? Casting directors of cinema and TV films frequently select actors to play parts for which they look 'right'. In 1946 Berelson and Salter in a study of stereotypes in fiction found that villains tended to be dark and swarthy whereas heroes tended to be blond. One wonders to what extent these same prejudices apply today and to what degree they should really be termed 'prejudices' in the sense that this word implies prejudgments being made which have no validity. It could well be that in real life most heroes are blond.

Recently Shoemaker, South and Lowe (1973) found evidence that we do have stereotypic notions about the appearance criminals have. They concluded that,

> on the basis of our findings it would be plausible to assume
> that stereotypic conceptions of what a particular suspect
> should look like could influence the selection of 'the one who
> did it' by an eyewitness of a crime, particularly when that
> eyewitness did not have a good, clear look at the offender.

In this study fifty-four facial photographs of middle-aged, white
males were shown to audiences of students who were asked to
rate how likely the person was to have committed murder or
robbery or treason. The twelve photographs which received the
most extreme rankings were then shown to a second group of
audiences and each audience rated the portrayed individual for
his likelihood of having committed one of the crimes. Here significant differences were observed across photographs indicating
the employment of stereotypes. Further audiences were given
brief written accounts of ambiguously criminal incidents attached
to which was one of the twelve photographs. The extent of attributed guilt was found to be significantly influenced by which of
the photographs was attached. These results were obtained (with
rather poor methodology) in artificial circumstances, but the
processes which they claim to highlight are likely to be operative
in the real world. Buckhout (1974b) describes an experiment
conducted by Allport in which observers briefly looked at a
drawing of several people sitting or standing in a subway train.
One of the people in this scene was black and a white man near
to him was holding an open, cut-throat razor. When later asked
to describe the scene, 50 per cent of the observers reported that
the razor had been in the hand of the black man. Buckhout
believes that, 'most people file away some stereotypes on the
basis of which they make perceptual judgements; such stereotypes not only fit in with prejudices but they are also tools for
making decisions more efficiently.'

VALIDITY

The question as to what extent physical appearances are valid
indices of behavioural characteristics has been examined for
many decades and was popular even before the advent of psy-

chology as we know it. A great number of studies have been conducted in this area but it is likely that many of those finding no significant relationships have remained unpublished (a frequent occurrence in the behavioural sciences). However, whether existing stereotypes are correct or not is largely irrelevant to the role they can play in person recognition and description. As Liggett (1974) points out, it does not matter to what extent these biases, expectancies and prejudices have any validity, what matters is if people believe that such relationships exist and if people use them. (If they do so believe then a number of important and often self-fulfilling prophecies follow.)

Secord (1958) gave a brief verbal personality account of two imaginary characters to a group of subjects. One of the characters was described as 'warmhearted and honest', the other 'ruthless and brutal'. The subjects were required to give some indication of the appearance they expected the characters to have by rating on seven-point scales each of 32 facial (and hair) characteristics. For 25 of these 32 features the ratings were found to be significantly different as a function of the personality accounts. Secord noted that for the majority of those characteristics which differentiated between the two descriptions the 'warmhearted and honest' person was rated as being average (e.g. average width of nose) whereas the 'ruthless and brutal' individual was judged as having abnormal features (for example, the observers accorded to him either an extremely narrow nose or an extremely wide one). It seems that the observers in Secord's study were employing a stereotype that has frequently come to the present second author's notice in his study of the psychological significance of facial deformity, namely that the general public take abnormality of appearance to be indicative of abnormality of personality and likely behaviour. In his book entitled *Stigma*, Goffman (1963) notes that this term was originated by the Greeks who burnt or cut signs into the body to signify that the bearer was a slave, a criminal or a traitor. Goffman believes that today we often take abnormality of appearance to indicate not only that there is *something* abnormal about the person but that such people are *totally* abnormal. We take strange appearance to be synonymous with strange personality, character or likely behaviour. Goffman observes that society frequently assigns to a person with a peculiar appearance the role of someone 'quite thoroughly bad, or dangerous, or weak'. MacGregor, Abel, Bryt, Lauer and Weissmann (1953) showed photographs of persons, some with facial anomalies, to non-disfigured persons who were asked to describe the photographed individuals. One was of a man with narrow, deep-set eyes, a prominent nose, buck teeth, a receding pointed chin, a small forehead and lop ears. It was not mentioned that in fact he was of high intelligence and an executive in a large company. Descriptions of the man such as the following were often voiced: 'He looks like a maniac. He's a dope addict. He's mean and small. He is in a gang. He has a desire to kill.' MacGregor *et al.* concluded that, 'facial features led respondents not only to impute to these patients personality traits considered socially unacceptable, but to assign to them roles and statuses on an inferior social level.' For our present purposes the studies cited above indicate that people will both deduce behavioural and attitudinal propensities from a seen face and will also generate likely facial features from behavioural data.

Thornton (1939) selected from the files of the Nebraska State Penitentiary the case records of twenty criminals, deliberately avoiding seeing the photographs of the criminals until this selection had been made. Since he was going to ask people to indicate which crime the particular individual had committed by looking at a portrait photograph of a criminal, Thornton wisely wanted to avoid selecting criminals whose photographs matched his own stereotype. (Thus this researcher avoided the possibility of a biased selection of photographs about which observers might agree solely because the experimenter had specially selected the photographs in the first place.) These photographs were shown one at a time to a large audience who were required to say which of four crimes they thought each photographed individual had committed. The observers were correct more often than was accountable by chance factors alone but they were by no means overwhelmingly so. Thus Thornton concluded that, 'the subjects showed some ability to gain from photographs cues which aided them slightly in judging what crime a man had committed, but this effect is so slight that for practicable purposes it is negligible.'

Hurwitz, Wiggins and Jones (1975) found that personality traits are readily attributed to facial photographs in a consistent manner and Hochberg and Galper (1974) showed how intention can be attributed as a function of physiognomy. The latter authors concluded that, 'physiognomy does affect the attribution of behavioural intentions and perceivers can reliably attribute intentions on the basis of still photographs of faces.' Unfortunately in this study, though inter-observer agreement was found, there was no attempt to see if such judgments had any real predictive validity. Bradshaw (1969) using schematic faces, as did Brunswik (1956), observed that, 'people acted in a fairly regular and statistically predictable way in attributing personality characteristics to these.' He found, for example, that when the eyes were placed 'up' on the schematic face, such a face was regarded as significantly more trustworthy than the same face on which the eyes were placed lower. Roll and Verinis (1971) observed that different hair styles on the same face led to different judgments and Chapman (1975) observed fairly high consistency across raters of schematic faces (which varied only in the vertical positioning of eyes, nose, mouth) for judgments of intelligence, happiness and likeableness. The existence of such effects may have implications for procedures like that of photofit (described in Chapter 4) though Bradshaw and McKenzie (1971) found less marked effects in their replications of Bradshaw's earlier study.

What the studies mentioned in the above paragraph were unable to do was to decide whether such stereotypes have any validity. Many years ago Hull (1928) collected forty facial photographs of female students who were all inter-acquainted. 'True' character judgments were obtained by the friends of each photographed individual completing a number of rating scales whilst looking at the photograph of the person. High inter-judge agreement was found here. Next the photographs were rated by people who were unacquainted with the photographed individuals. Again high inter-judge agreement was noted. However, when the 'true' and 'stranger' ratings were compared for each of the photographs the resulting correlations were very low (save for 'beauty' and 'intelligence'). Thus though the strangers agreed upon their expectancies about the photographed individuals these were not the same as those held by people who knew the individuals concerned. Cleeton and Knight (1924) noted similar effects to those found by Hull, plus the existence of only low correlations between judgments of individuals' character attributes and twenty-eight measured aspects of their faces and heads.

Secord, Dukes and Bevan (1954) found observers to agree largely upon the personality characteristics they expected· photographed individuals to possess. The highest agreements were for judgments of 'cheerful appearance, sense of humour, self-confident, intelligent, determined, likeable, honest', and the lowest agreements were for 'expressive face, studious, indifferent, shy, meek'. Another group of judges displayed very high inter-agreement for judgments of physiognomy, the highest agreements being for 'age, eyebrows (heavy vs. light), lips (full vs. thin), face-width, mouth-curvature', and the lowest for 'set of jaw, distance between eyes'. (Those working on the man-machine recognition systems described in Chapter 4 might note this work.) Having performed a form of cluster analysis Secord *et al.* concluded, 'That impressions of physiognomy and personality are significantly associated has been amply demonstrated', and they noted that the observers were frequently unable to verbalize concerning the bases for their ratings of personality. It is interesting to note that in this study the vast majority of significant associations between physiognomic cues and personality traits were for facial attributes which are strongly indicative of emotional feeling e.g. 'mouth curvature, facial tension', even though the photographs were selected on the basis of 'avoiding those with easy recognizable emotional expressions'. The aforementioned two cues accounted for 77 per cent of the significant associations whereas the facial attributes which do not vary so much in emotion were not often consistently used by the various observers in making their judgments of personality.

The finding of Secord *et al.* that mouth curvature was an important factor in their experiment ties in with the observation of Ellis, Shepherd and Davies (1975) that when using the photo-fit method of reconstructing faces (see Chapter 4) subjects were much poorer at selecting the correct mouth in the 'face absent' condition than in the 'face present' situation. Though only a limited number of faces was used by Ellis *et al.* this suggests the possibility that observers may not retain in memory an accurate, fixed impression of the mouth since its appearance is so variable both as a function of emotion and of speech.

Having needed to resort to cluster analysis, Secord *et al.* stated that, 'These results suggest that the conventional ele-mentalizing used by psychologists is simply inappropriate.' Unfortunately Secord's study offers no information concerning the validity of the observed stereotypes. Recently Terry and Snider (1972) showed photographs of students to an audience unacquainted with the students. The observers were asked to say for each photograph whether the student was likely to be a member of (i) a scholastic society, or (ii) an athletic club, or (iii) an extra-curricular society, or (iv) none of these. High agreement was noted between the judgments and these were veridical. Thus, a perceived individual's appearance can influ-ence a perceiver's expectations of how such a person will behave or did behave.

One does not know to what extent Deputy Assistant Com-missioner David Powis was aware of the research which had been conducted in this area but he advised policemen to observe in court persons in custody for the theft or unlawful taking of motor vehicles to 'see to which category they belong. This will help you to slant your mind to the general type of person you must watch for when patrolling.' It is certainly not possible to say that such advice is worthless but it may be that such advice can be misguided and productive of errors of commission. The important thing is to be able to gauge how useful it is and similarly to be able to know to what extent stereotypic notions play a role in person recognition situa-tions. Bruner, Shapiro and Tagiuri (1958) have reminded us that,

It is a truism that the acts performed by people are not independent of one another – a man who steals is likely to lie as well. The fact of consistency of behaviour, the backbone of personality theories, is represented in the language by which people are commonly described. It is characteristic of words like 'honest' or 'clever' that they do more than denote specific acts of a person. Indeed, they summarize or package certain consistencies of behaviour.

ATTRACTIVENESS

Physical attractiveness is a variable which is currently receiving much attention from psychologists (in the experimental sense!) and research suggests that we might not expect persons having certain appearances to be involved in crime and that we might not be inclined to pick them out in 'an identification parade or from memory. The converse may also be true. Do we tend at a later date to recognize only the attractive (or outstanding) strangers who were at the party a few weeks ago though at the time we saw the faces of all who were present? Doob and Kirshenbaum (1973) report a case in which a witness could remember little about a robber except that he was 'rather good looking'.

Cavior, Hayes and Cavior (1975) suggest that, 'low physical attractiveness contributes to careers of deviancy' and in 1941 Monahan noted that,

> even social workers accustomed to dealing with all types
> often find it difficult to think of a normal, pretty girl as
> being guilty of a crime. Most people, for some inexplicable
> reason, think of crime in terms of abnormality of
> appearance and I must say that beautiful women are not
> often convicted.

Jones and Hirschberg (1975) found that an individual's facial attractiveness had an effect on how threatening other people judged that person to be. They observed that the more attractive a person's face the less threatening was the individual believed to be. It has already been mentioned that film and advertising directors have for years chosen as the 'baddy' a small, ugly, weasel-looking individual and as the 'goody' a tall, attractive, clean-cut type. Landy and Aronson (1969) found, in a simulated setting, that the appearance of the defendant had a significant effect upon 'jurors' decisions about the length of prison sentence that should be given. The unattractive defendant was sentenced far more severely for a given crime than a defendant with an attractive character and appearance. In part of this study the character of the victim of the crime was also varied and it was found that the defendant tended to receive a more severe sentence if the victim was attractive. Sigall and Ostrove (1974) varied only the physical attractiveness of the defendant and did not also concomitantly vary the character descriptions as Landy had done. Here again the attractiveness of the (female) defendant had an effect upon the sentence given. However, the effect of attractiveness interacted with the nature of the crime. That is, as expected from previous findings, an attractive burglar received a less severe sentence than an unattractive burglar (6 vs. 9 years), but an attractive swindler received a stiffer sentence than an unattractive swindler. (Possible reasons for this are provided in Bull (1974).) Interestingly 'judges' given no information about the defendant's beauty attributed significantly greater physical attractiveness to her as a swindler than as a burglar.

Efran (1974) also examined the effect of physical appearance on the judgment of guilt and the severity of recommended punishment in a simulated jury task. As in many psychological experiments the people who took part in the experiment were students who may or may not behave in the same way as would other members of the population. Over 100 people filled in a questionnaire and this survey revealed that (a) only 21 per cent believed that a defendant's character and previous history should not influence juror's decision, whereas (b) over 93 per cent believed that the defendant's physical appearance should not bias these decisions. A further sixty-six students received written details of an example of alleged cheating during an examination and they were required to rate how likely it was that the person mentioned had been cheating and the extent of punishment that should be given. Two-thirds of the 'jurors' also received a photograph of the defendant and these were also required as their last task to rate the defendant for physical attractiveness. For each of these 'jurors' the photograph was of an opposite sexed individual. Efran found for female defendants that the more physically attractive individuals were judged to be significantly less guilty and to merit milder punishment than the unattractive female defendants. No effect of physical attractiveness was apparent for the male defendants. This difference could be due to the possibility that the physical attractiveness of male defendants does not play a role in such settings with female 'jurors', or to the possibility that the male defendants did not differ much in their level of physical attractiveness. This latter suggestion is supported by the attractiveness ratings. Whereas the female defendants did significantly differ in the attractiveness ratings they received the male defendants did not. Whether the male defendants did not in reality differ much in attractiveness, or whether the allegation that they were cheats reduced the good-looking ones' attractiveness for the female jurors is not known. However, the male photographs which were used had been deemed to be significantly different in attractiveness in one of Efran's earlier studies.

Dion (1972) believes that good-looking people are seen as possessing more socially desirable traits than unattractive individuals. She found that the attractiveness of the photograph on a child's report card had an effect upon judgments of misbehaviour. Female students were given written details of a child's misbehaviour together with a photograph which was supposed to be of the child. The description of the misdeed was always exactly the same and the only thing that varied was that some students saw a photograph of an attractive child and some saw a photograph of an unattractive child. It was found that the students suggested more lenient treatment for the attractive child. Those who saw a photograph of an attractive child said that the misbehaviour was likely to be only a temporary thing whereas those with a photograph of an unattractive individual frequently said that they believed it likely that the child was often naughty, was anti-social, and should be severely punished.

In Dion's study inexperienced students were employed as the assessors but in a similar study by Clifford and Walster (1973) experienced teachers were shown a nursery child's report card to which was attached a photograph. The teachers were asked to rate the child and it was found that although the report card always said exactly the same thing the more attractive the child in the photograph (established by prior study) the more favourable were the teachers' evaluations of IQ, peer relationships, likely future educational accomplishments and parents' attitudes towards school. Rich (1975) again used as subjects experienced teachers who were given a child's report card plus a photograph. The teachers were asked to say how likely it was that the child had been the naughty one in class and if so, what punishment should be given. As would be expected, the nature of the report card greatly influenced the teachers' decisions. If the report card was good then little punishment was advocated. However, if the report card was bad the teachers who had the unattractive male photographs were more inclined to suggest harsher punishment. These three studies illustrate that the physical attractiveness stereotype may operate even in the world of young school-children. (Bull and Stevens (in press) found similar effects upon experienced teachers' ratings of an undergraduate's essay.) It is important to note here that not only may we judge an individual's likely anti-social behaviour by the way he looks but that in behaving towards children in this way we may create in them certain predispositions which then result in the existence of some self-fulfilling prophecies. Physically attractive children may receive more positive attention and support when they are young and because of this they develop greater social skills and self-confidence. As a consequence they become attractive in more than just the physical sense and in adulthood such people may indeed be more worth approaching and be more successful than physically unattractive individuals who have not developed such attributes. It seems likely to be a widely held stereotype that physically attractive individuals are not so inclined to do unpleasant or anti-social things. Thus, when in doubt we might hesitate to pick such a person out from an identification parade, from mugshots and from memory in general. On the other hand, if a witness did get a good view of someone whom he was later required to recognize then it has been found that attractive faces are recognized better than unattractive ones (Cross, Cross and Daly, 1971). Shepherd and Ellis (1973) found that faces both high and low on attractiveness were better recognized than those of medium attractiveness and they suggest that the findings of Cross *et al.* may merely have been a function of the fact that in the study by Cross *et al.* there was no control over the time that the subjects initially spent looking at each face. Shepherd and Ellis argue that if the subjects spent a greater time viewing the more attractive faces then the superior recognition of these faces is not at all surprising. However, Cross *et al.* (1971) comment that if anything their observers spent the least time looking at the attractive faces.

BODY-BUILD

Variations in body-build have also been found to lead to stereo-typic expectancies. Brunswik (1956) noted that with the face kept constant differences in stature led to significantly different judgments of personality. Lerner and Korn (1972) observed that differences in body-build reliably had effects upon the judg-ments children made about individuals. Both these authors and Staffieri (1972) note that as a child develops, the imposition of stereotypes will shape his behaviour and that this might result in the stereotypes actually becoming valid (i.e. if a child looks 'naughty' and people act accordingly towards him might he therefore believe that this is his role in life?). Powell, Tutton and Stewart (1974) feel that, 'a socio-expectational model of the relationships between behaviour and physique is plausible.'

Some studies have shown that it is possible to validly judge a person's occupation solely from their photograph. Litterer (1933) observed this as did Gahagan (1933), but Landis and Phelps (1928) did not. Child (1936) noted inter-judge agreement con-cerning the occupations of pictured individuals and these judgments remained stable in a retest three months later.

The implication of all the studies mentioned in this chapter is that observers' recall of individuals will be a function not only of what they actually perceived at the time of the relevant incident but also of what their stereotypic notions suggest to them. Furthermore, some researchers believe that stereotypes can have an influence not only on the nature of recall but also at the time of perception. Stritch and Secord (1956) stated that their 'results suggest that personality impressions formed from the photographs act as organizing factors in the perception of physiognomic traits.' More research is certainly needed on this particular hypothesis but it does seem likely that when the sighting of an individual is incomplete (or memory fades) the observer will add factors, and these probably will be a function of his stereotypes and expectancies. The publication *Science and the Police* (from the British Association for the Advancement of Science) stated that, 'There is a tendency to fill in gaps in remembrance, even of those parts of a happening where what actually occurred has been forgotton.' Freedman and Haber (1974) have suggested that, 'The organizational properties of perceptual memory are important determinants of the adequacy of that memory' and that their study provided 'evidence that recognition memory is aided by perceiver-elicited organizations imposed on the material to be remembered', that is, the schema-generated perceptions we discussed in Chapter 2. These very often *non-conscious* effects can influence the judgments and recall of witnesses. Razran (1938, 1950) has found that even the type of surname added to a photograph can have a significant effect upon judgments made of the portrayed person.

In a series of experiments presently being conducted in our department by Clive Hollin some evidence has been found to support Wall's (1965) observations that witnesses often infer the presence of one physical feature from their recall of the observed person's possession of another. A person entered a lecture to search for a briefcase and after walking around the room the lecturer asked him to leave. In the first of such incidents the 'target' person was blond, with green eyes and a fair complexion. The eyewitnesses descriptions of the target person were very accurate for hair colour, 93 per cent of the witnesses reporting that the hair was blond. However, of this 93 per cent almost half described the person as having blue eyes, whereas only 7 per cent correctly said green. (Fourteen per cent incorrectly reported other colours and the remainder did not mention eye colour at all.) Of those who reported blond hair three quarters correctly reported the target person as having a fair complexion. Thus the proportion of the observers which indicated that the target person had blond hair, a fair complexion and *blue* eyes was 36 per cent. In the second incident, with a different audience, the target person had dark hair, grey eyes and a light complexion. All the observers in this part of the study described correctly the target person's hair colour. However, over half of them incorrectly reported the eye colour as being brown and none of them correctly reported it as being grey. Forty-four per cent correctly reported a fair complexion whereas 56 per cent reported the target person as having a dark complexion. Thus the proportion of the observers who reported that the target person had dark hair, *brown* eyes and a *dark* complexion was 44 per cent. Hollin takes these effects of blond hair incorrectly implying blue eyes, and dark hair suggesting brown eyes and a dark complexion to indicate that witnesses fill in gaps in their recall by employing stereotypes or known population norms. Sometimes such confabulation will be correct (perhaps even most times if the stereotype has validity) but on some occasions it will lead to inaccurate descriptions being given. The high proportion of witnesses correctly reporting the hair colour suggests, as is obvious, that this physical attribute is more readily perceived than eye colour or type of complexion and therefore it should carry more weight in real-life circumstances where descriptions are required. Unfortunately, hair colour is more easily changed than is eye colour and so even though details of the target person's hair may be more reliably reported they are not so fixed aspects of a person as are other attributes such as eye colour and type of complexion.

That stereotypic factors play a role in person perception and recollection has been amply demonstrated and it is likely that these effects operate when a witness is unsure and yet is being pressed either implicitly or explicitly to say something. However, most of the studies cited were conducted in the laboratory and the possible extent of most of these influences in real-life settings remains to be investigated.

4 Identification by means of face

While we hope to show in other chapters that recognition of persons can be achieved by remembering such things as voice, gait, clothing and mannerisms, by far the most powerful means of recognition is by perceiving, storing and retrieving aspects of facial configuration. This may be due to the fact that the face is the most salient feature of a person's being, and indeed, quantification of various aspects of social interactions have confirmed the notion that people look mainly at each others faces (Argyle, 1969). While Harmon (1973) believes that 'determining how one recognises a face is probably an intractable problem at present', and although Knapp (1972) suggests that 'the face is the researcher's nightmare', none the less we will attempt to set out how the problem of face identification has been approached and what progress has been achieved. As mentioned in Chapter 2 memory is usually measured by means of either recognition or recall. Most laboratory studies of facial memory have employed recognition, but lately a few have employed recall measures by means of photofit, artist drawings and identikit. Both types of measure will be discussed below. A crucial first step in the application of psychological findings to law enforcement procedures would be to clarify just how a face is processed and how it is stored, and it is with this that we begin.

SINGLE FEATURE SALIENCY

Faces are complex patterns which comprise a number of intra-facial sub-patterns (Ellis, 1975). It would seem advantageous to examine just which part, or parts, of a face are scrutinized most during inspection and then try to relate inspection intensity and duration to later recognition.

Ontogenetically it would appear that very young children show differential fixation to eyes. Fantz, Fagan and Miranda (1975), and Caron, Caron, Caldwell and Weiss (1973), together with Gibson (1969), showed that infants seem to learn to attend to people's eyes before they attend to their mouths. By and large psychology has shown that that which is learned or developed first is used most, or best, in later adulthood. Thus a prediction would be that adults should also fixate eyes more than other parts of the face. This is precisely what is observed when one monitors the eye movements of a person looking at a face (Munn, 1961; Yarbus, 1967; Zusne, 1970). If fixation frequency, or duration, can be used to indicate parameters of facial processing, and it is shown that eyes and mouth are the features most looked at, then perhaps those features which best aid recognition are precisely the eyes and the mouth. An early study by Howells (1938), however, found that covering the lower part of the face during initial presentation was more deleterious to recognition than covering the upper part of the face, thus going against both the ontogenetic and the 'frequency and type of fixation' predictions. Later research does, however, support these predictions because Goldstein and Mackenberg (1966), testing school-children, found just the opposite result to Howells (1938), and Laughery, Alexander and Lane (1971), using a technique woefully under-used by psychologists, showed that the prediction was substantiated. The latter authors simply asked their subjects to say how they were doing the task of remembering faces! They said that the features which best aided recognition were eyes, nose, mouth, lips, chin, hair and ears, in that order. Friedman, Reed and Carterette (1971), using schematic faces, elicited a similar ordering of saliency, which was nose, eyes, forehead then mouth. While there are slight differences in the two orderings the general point is that eyes are given high saliency rating, and although the studies by Ellis, Shepherd and Davies (1975) are somewhat ambiguous with respect to mouth-eye importance in photo-fit construction, additional support for eye saliency comes from studies by McKelvie (1976a), again using schematic faces, and, in a study to be discussed below, Fisher and Cox (1975) clearly indicate that the eyes are the most salient facial feature in the recognition of photographs of famous people.

According to McKelvie (1976a) the weight of evidence in favour of eyes may explain poorer recognition in such situations as inversion, because as Yin (1969) suggests, the major problem with an upside-down face is apparently its loss of expression and, as we will see, expression plays a role in facial recognition. Further, the eyes are the chief source of such expression (Ekman, Friesen and Ellsworth, 1972; Liggett, 1974). Because the eyes and mouth are more 'expression carrying' it is possible that they attract more attention and as a result people learn to differentiate these more, and thus provide more labels for these aspects of facial features. Whatever the reason for the greater fixation of some parts rather than others, the possibility of greater differentiation, and therefore availability of labels ought to be capitalized upon.

FEATURES IN COMBINATION

Over and above features in isolation there are also features in combination. As was indicated above in the studies by Laughery *et al.* (1971) and by Friedman *et al.* (1971), when subjects are asked to order facial features in terms of salience for recognition a fairly clear order appeared. However, Friedman *et al.* found that such a saliency ranking did not completely predict face recognition performance. Changing one feature rated low (e.g. forehead) did not produce greater decrement in recognition performance than changing a feature rated high (e.g. nose). Friedman *et al.* also noted that though observers were quite good at noting that two faces were different they could rarely specify which feature had changed. This strongly implicates perception of pattern rather than of specific individual features. Perhaps after all, the whole is greater than the sum of the parts, and indeed most of the subjects in Laughery *et al.*'s study rated 'General Structure' as *the* most important determiner of later recognition.

Several years ago Fisher and Cox (1975) examined feature

73

saliency in recognition, and the possibility of a facial gestalt. By progressively increasing the amount of a facial photograph observable to the viewer, either horizontally or vertically, they were able to work out which were the most important features for recognition and whether two features were multiplicative rather than merely additive in their effect. They found that the upper features of human faces convey appreciably more information for recognition than lower features. This agrees with, among others, Goldstein and Mackenberg (1966) and Nash (1969), but is at odds with Howells (1938). Fisher and Cox found that the eyes contributed most to identification, but they were careful to stress that revealed features below the level of the eyes were sufficiently informative to allow recognition of famous people in 64 per cent of cases. Over and above specific feature saliency, Fisher and Cox stressed features in combination because they found that lower parts of the face contribute approximately 15 per cent more information when presented within the context of upper features than when presented alone (i.e. with no upper features of the face). A configurational aspect is also suggested by the fact that the addition of eyes produces the greatest increase in recognition, suggesting that eyes are the most important facial feature for recognition, *but* only 12 per cent of subjects recognized the face when the eyes were presented in isolation. This suggests that the importance of eye detail is enhanced considerably by the immediately surrounding context.

It ought perhaps to be pointed out in passing that even with very familiar photographs false recognition occurred, e.g. being presented with the upper hairline of Emanuel Shinwell often caused false identification responses of 'Malcolm Muggeridge' who was not present.

PERCEPTUAL GESTALT

This emphasis upon the role of the interrelationships between features has been forcibly made by among others Liggett (1974), who points out perspicaciously that facial proportions and features, but not their patterning, can change a great deal in childhood yet we can often recognize a child we have not seen for many years. This observation was also made by Arnheim

(1949) when he argued that the whole structure of a face rather than the sum of its parts determines expression. Yin (1969) noted that in facial recognition tasks his subjects 'attempted to get a general impression of the whole picture' rather than search for some distinguishing feature and Tversky (1969), while finding a suggestion of additivity of various features, still maintained that 'interactive or Gestalt effects are important'. Recourse to everyday impressions, and the logic of finite numbers, renders it obvious that few faces have outstanding single features and thus single feature searches might not prove efficient in most cases. While all faces are unique to some degree none the less each component of this 'uniqueness' will be present in innumerable other faces. Given this consideration, Caron *et al.* (1973) may be correct when they say that we may learn to perceive and discriminate faces in a wholistic way, and it is further possible that an observed individual's facial features may not always originate in perception as isolated elements, features may 'differentiate in configurational relationships', i.e. we may see the whole before we can see the parts.

Direct evidence for perceptual gestalt effects has been given by Homa, Haver and Schwartz (1976). Their initial orientating interest stemmed from work in verbal memory and perception where it has been shown that the perceptibility of any letter in a word is greater than the perceptibility of that same letter shown in isolation, or the same letters scrambled to form unpronounceable words (Baron and Thurston, 1973; Reicher, 1969). Homa *et al.* wished to see if this word superiority effect (WSE) would generalize to the perception of visual forms, particularly faces. They addressed the problem of whether, in general, the perceptibility of the constituent parts of a face would be enhanced when those parts were ordered or organized in some well defined pattern such as a normal face pattern. Homa *et al.* presented scrambled faces, ordinary faces and features in isolation. The features to be perceived were eyes, nose and mouth. The parallel here with the WSE studies is clear: the single letter is equivalent to a single face feature, scrambled letters are equivalent to scrambled faces, and normal words equivalent to normal faces. The word superiority effect would be reproduced with visual forms if it could be shown that any feature embedded in a normal face pattern was perceived with greater accuracy than when that feature appeared either by itself or in an anomalous face. The basic procedure was to show subjects a card on which was either an ordinary face, a scrambled face or a single feature, for a very short duration via a tachistiscope (a machine which can present visual displays for very brief periods of time), then to present a visual mask (which served to obliterate the face or feature previously shown) and finally to ask subjects to recognize which feature had been presented from a card containing that feature (e.g. nose) plus another four distractors (noses). Three different experiments were run but only the general results will be discussed here. Across all three experiments perception of single feature and face stimuli were consistently superior to scrambled faces. For our purposes, in terms of face perception, the interesting comparison is between scrambled and normal faces, and the finding that subjects were much more accurate with normal faces suggests that the perceptibility of constituent features is enhanced when these features are arranged within a well defined pattern. Disruption of scanning strategies habitually used by subjects cannot explain the result because the scrambled faces were always organized from top to bottom in an invariant order, and the subjects had ample learning (familiarization) opportunities. Homa *et al.* conclude, 'hypothesis of a perceptual Gestalt must be seriously entertained for well defined form stimuli, where a perceptual Gestalt is defined as the enhanced perceptibility of the constituent parts due to the general form class of the stimulus.' Another important finding, in terms of the work we have quoted above on priority in facial feature scanning, is that Homa *et al.* found that eyes and mouths were much better perceived than were noses when either normal or scrambled faces were used, but not when single feature displays were used. This suggests that when subjects are confronted with a total face, attentional demands are diverted to eyes and mouth with a consequential decrease in processing of the nose, and hence its later, poorer recall or recognition.

Allport, as in so many things, may have said it all before when, in 1937, he stated that features in isolation are not nearly as intelligible as patterns and yet it is obvious that in some way the total pattern is composed of these very same features. In terms of the ideas developed in Chapter 2, based on Chomsky's surface and deep structure notions, it is noteworthy that Galper and Hochberg (1971) suggest, in the light of their research findings, that it is possible that faces are remembered by a combination of configurational patterns and single specific cues. Where a face has an outstanding feature (surface structure feature) this will be remembered and greatly aid recognition, but when this is not so, noting the patterning (deep structure features) will prove more useful. It is a fact that some faces are more memorable than others. Cross *et al.* (1971) stated that the differences in the memorability of individual faces was a notable result of their studies and the continuum of memorability was a function of the ordinariness of the face, the most ordinary being the least memorable.

FACIAL ATTRIBUTES

If it is really facial patterns we ought to be investigating then perhaps it ought to be facial qualities other than features which should be researched and scaled. Little investigation has been made concerning facial attributes but that which has been performed is instructive. Cross *et al.* (1971) examined the role of beauty in recognition and found that faces initially rated high in beauty were subsequently better recognized. While this study is a clear case of an attribute predicting future recognition, Cross *et al.* failed to control for inspection time and thus they were unable to rule out the possibility that subjects merely looked longer at good-looking stimuli and thus better coded that face, there being some evidence of better coding with increased viewing time (Ellis, 1975). However, a subjective impression on the part of Cross *et al.* was that the good-looking faces (which eventually were better recalled) were actually processed for a shorter time than the other faces.

Pleasantness is another attribute of a face which has been shown to influence memorability positively. Peters (1917) obtained a rating of pleasantness from subjects after they had attempted to recognize a face on a recognition trial. Pleasant faces were remembered best, low rated faces were memorized next best, and medium rated faces were remembered worst of all. This type of curvilinear relationship is a frequent finding in psychology, and in terms of face recognition seems to be reproducible. Shepherd and Ellis (1973) had faces independently rated for attractiveness by subjects who did not take part in the memory phase of the experiment, and then they compared the recognition of these differently rated faces at various times after the initial viewing. A curvilinear relationship was evident at delayed recognitions of thirty-five days. At this delay the top third (most attractive) and the bottom third (least attractive) rated faces were best recognized, with medium attractive faces being poorest. Shepherd and Ellis interpret the findings in terms of arousal theory: high and low attractive faces are more arousing than those of medium attractiveness and this in turn produces stronger memory traces (e.g. Kleinsmith and Kaplan, 1963). This arousal explanation seems rather weak, however, and essentially *post hoc* and the results of a recent study by Fleishman, Buckley, Klosinsky, Smith and Tuck (1976) only serve to cloud the issue. These researchers found that the superiority of both attractive and unattractive faces over 'neutral' faces occurred two hours after presentation, whereas Shepherd and Ellis failed to get this effect at a six-day lag. Thus Shepherd and Ellis obtained an effect of high and low attractiveness at thirty-five days but not at six days, whereas Fleishman *et al.* obtained the effect at two hours. This conflicting finding would not be predicted from a simple arousal hypothesis. The work performed by Bower and Karlin (1974) concerning depth of processing discussed above may offer a more valid explanation, and the possibility of differential labelling of attractive, non-attractive and neutral faces should be explored.

Expression could be another very important attribute in facial recognition. One of the many problems of using schematic faces in face research is their limited capacity to portray expression, an ability which real faces possess to a high degree. Liggett (1974) believes that the human face is 'man's most varied attribute' and this variability comes not only from differences in shape but also from differences in mobility, there being over 100 distinguishable muscles in each face. If it is true that it is this interrelationship between facial features that most aids our recognition of others (Liggett, 1974) and if, as Stritch and Secord (1956) found, alterations of a physiognomic attribute in otherwise identical photographs of a face will induce perception of change in other facial characteristics, then since facial expression involves changes in the distance between facial features (and in the size of the features themselves, viz. the eyes and mouth), one might expect facial expression to play a role in recognition. The problem with expression is that because any individual can change his expression it may be less than helpful in a diagnosis of how best to improve eyewitness performance. It is of little use knowing that expression plays an important part in face memory if in fact expressions can be altered at will. Persons under stress, such as when performing criminal episodes or, more familiarly when performing difficult skills, show facial expressions which are not present when they are not under such performance pressures.

One expression that has been studied in terms of facial recognition is smiling. Galper and Hochberg (1971) studied the performance of subjects who were shown either a smiling or an unsmiling face and were then tested on recognition with the same face posed in the alternative expression. Five days elapsed between viewing and recognition and it was found that the change in expression caused a decrement in performance. It is unfortunate that these researchers failed to build in a control condition which could allow us to compare differential recognition of faces initially and eventually seen in either a smiling or non-smiling pose. Sorce and Campos (1974) served to consolidate the importance of expression change for recognition by showing that the greater the difference between a face's expression on initial viewing and later recognition testing the poorer was recognition performance.

Smiling could be subsumed under an attribute theory and should be helpful to recognition if we could ensure similarity between viewing and identification – an identification parade would allow this by virtue of being 'live'. That smiling could be attribute-based is supported by Thornton (1943), who found that smiling faces were judged as more honest.

CHANGED APPEARANCE

Allied to expression is the possibility of poor memory for a person who alters his appearance by, for example, donning glasses or a wig, shaving off a moustache or beard, etc. Very little work has been done on this transformation parameter, although Patterson at Cambridge is conducting some relevant experiments. McKelvie (1976a) indicated that one of the central issues in the current debate about human memory is the nature of the representation of any given stimulus and specifically, what aspects of the stimulus are processed and in what form they are stored. One approach to the tricky problem of storage format is to investigate what transformations have a detrimental affect on recognition. McKelvie (1976a) presented twenty-seven photographs of faces for inspection with or without transformations (that is, eyes or mouth could be masked) and tested for recognition with or without the same or different transformations. Subjects made more errors when the eyes were masked. Subjects performed best when inspection and recognition involved the same facial transformation or non-transformation (i.e. inspecting an eye-masked face and recognizing a non eye-masked face produced many errors). This study also served to clarify the finding of Ellis *et al.* (1975) who, using two photographs, suggested that there were individual differences among faces in the extent to which eyes or mouth were more important for processing and remembering. McKelvie showed that masking the eyes always caused greater errors in recognition than masking the mouth.

SCANNING

So far, then, we have looked at possible facial features which may have important psychological implications for an understanding of how people perceive faces and go about recognizing them. In a real sense, however, these stimulus features only become important when they are being actively processed by the would-be recognizer. Thus, an important consideration for the psychology of person identification is the specification of the scanning strategies of people when confronted by a face, and their possible modifiability. One oblique approach to the elucidation of these encoding strategies is the use of inverted stimuli. Yin (1969) showed a five-fold increase in errors of recognition when the to-be-recognized face was presented upside down. This magnitude of error with inverted faces has also been found by Hochberg and Galper (1967), Scapinello and Yarmey (1970) and Yarmey (1971). The explanation seems to reside in a custo-mary, habitual strategy of perceiving being inappropriately employed when faces are inverted. Rock (1974) argued that inverting a face alters a number of spatial relationships with which we are extremely familiar, and such an alteration could therefore invalidate any well-established scanning strategy. The magnitude of the decrement in recognition with inverted faces compared to the decrement with inverted photographs of build-ings and other familiar objects suggests that facial scanning strategies are more over-learned or habitual. The interesting question then becomes can we improve recognition for inverted faces or more generally, can we change, modify and improve scanning strategies. If modifiability of such scanning strategies could be achieved this would have important implications for improving person recognition. Just such training effects have been demonstrated. Bradshaw and Wallace (1971) indicated that subjects very quickly learn to discriminate the features of an inverted face in a visual search task. As far as can be ascertained the usual face scanning pattern is (i) a top to bottom strategy, at least with schematic faces (Smith and Nielsen, 1970), coupled with (ii) a focusing on the eyes and mouth (Munn, 1961; Yarbus, 1967) and their relationship. The existence of such a consistent, well-grooved scanning pattern for looking at faces was supported by Noton and Stark (1971) who found that when given the same face to look at different people scanned it in the same way. Future research will have to provide solid evidence of exactly what strategies are employed, and how modifiable they are. A start has been made but much more work remains.

So far in this chapter we have looked at what could be called stimulus and individual factors in person recognition, that is the importance of feature like eyes, nose and mouth in accounting for the number and the length of fixations; features in combina-tion, the relationship between eyes nose and mouth; and facial attributes like smiling, 'honest', 'trustworthy' and 'attractive'. We then looked at the strategies which people employ while looking at a face, such as the top to bottom scan and we will later consider the emphasis that people place on the right side of the face when we consider the use of photo-fit in identification. For the moment, however, we will look more generally at face research as it applies to different groups of people.

INTRA- AND INTER-RACE FACIAL RECOGNITION

It is generally accepted that people of one race have great difficulty in recognizing people of another race. Malpass and Kravitz (1969) found that black and white subjects performed best with photographs of their own race, and this was replicated by Luce (1974) with different subjects and photographs and by Elliott, Wills and Goldstein (1973) who found that white observers were better at recognizing white faces than oriental faces. Chance, Goldstein and McBride (1975) showed that white subjects scored 68 per cent correct recognition of white faces, 55 per cent on black faces and only 45 per cent with oriental faces. Oriental faces also seem to create difficulty for black observers since Chance's black subjects scored 60 per cent correct recognition of black faces, 49 per cent on white faces but only 43 per cent with oriental faces. Thus it seems rather clear that recognition memory for faces is a complex interaction of both the observer and the observed, with identification being poorest when the race of the witness and the person observed does not match. Three explanations have been offered for the poor recognition of non-white faces by white subjects: (i) black faces may be inherently more difficult to recognize than white faces; (ii) whites have less familiarity with black faces and consequently have less opportunity to develop the necessary skills of perceiving and remembering other-race faces; (iii) certain forms of racial prejudice may predispose one race to process poorly faces of other races.

The 'inherently more difficult' hypothesis

This hypothesis has some appeal because there are features about white faces which suggest the possibility of greater individual discriminability relative to black faces (for example, white faces have a greater variety of hair colour and texture than negroes and also more variation in eye colouration). Unfortunately if this were the explanation for poor non-white face recognition one might expect black subjects to score exactly the same as white subjects when asked to recognize both black and white faces (i.e. black should do much better on white faces because of their greater individuality). However, the evidence is conflicting. The important question to ask is whether black subjects recognize black faces better than they can recognize white faces. The use of specifically black subjects recognizing black and white faces allows a direct investigation of the 'inherent difficulty' argument and in some studies where black subjects have been used as observers (Cross *et al.*, 1971; Malpass and Kravitz, 1969) they have been marginally better on white faces than black, but only marginally. This fact rules out a simple explanation in terms of best recognition for own race, and does in fact suggest that black faces are more difficult to discriminate. However, in a naturalistic cross-cultural setting Shepherd, Dėregowski and Ellis (1974) provided evidence for the 'best at own race' belief: black Rhodesian subjects were better at recognizing black faces and Scottish subjects were better at recognizing white faces. Luce (1974) has also shown that black people do have difficulty recognizing non-black faces, while Berger (1969) using a film sequence rather than still photographs also found this to be the case.

While some evidence exists that it is not necessarily the case that whites always have difficulty recognizing black faces (Galper, 1973, see below under 'prejudice hypothesis'), in light of the weight of evidence it could reasonably be argued that there would be differences in reliability between black and white eyewitnesses if the criminal was not of the same race as the witness, and this would seem not to be due to the inherently more difficult faces of one race or another. Goldstein, the chief researcher into the question of whether some races are inherently more difficulty to distinguish than others, in a paper presented to the Midwestern Psychological Association (1975b), investigated whether the folklore that 'all orientals look alike' had any basis in reality. He argued that if oriental faces were more homogeneous than white faces such a common belief would have some support. In the light of four experiments which basically involved comparing pairs of white and pairs of oriental faces he concluded that there was no justification for the belief that oriental faces were more homogeneous than white faces. Goldstein and Chance (1976), in the published version of Goldstein's first experiment, supported this contention.

The 'differential familiarity' hypothesis

This hypothesis would again appear intuitively to be a fairly good bet, but once again the psychological research does not totally support it. The evidence does not show that the greater the social interaction with black communities the greater the powers of recognition of non-white faces by white subjects. Luce (1974) did not find any significant difference between subjects who lived in mixed neighbourhoods and those who did not. Malpass and Kravitz (1969) elicted information on environmental lifestyle via questionnaire in their experiment and again failed to find any relationship between the amount of interracial contact and the ability to recognize other-race faces. These two negative studies have been supported by Berger (1969) and by Billig and Milner (1976), but differential familiarity could explain the study of Shepherd *et al.* (1974) discussed above, and Goldstein (1975b) and Goldstein and Chance (1976) favour this explanation.

One of the strongest pieces of evidence that differential familiarity has an effect in other-race face recognition comes from a study by Lavrakas, Buri and Mayzner (1976) who show that quantity and quality of experience related significantly to recognition performance. They point out, however, that quality is by far the more important factor. They say, 'Being white and actually having black friends was found to be more positively related to recognition of black faces than merely having grown up in an integrated neighbourhood or having gone to school with blacks.'

The 'racial attitude' hypothesis

This hypothesis has some good psychological evidence in its favour. We argued in Chapters 2 and 3 that we tend to see what we expect or want to see, and a great deal of evidence exists that prejudiced persons tend to view the world in terms of preconceived stereotypes. For instance, people who are prejudiced against blacks will have a preconceived visual stereotype that *all* blacks have curly hair, thick lips, wide noses, etc. There is a fair amount of evidence which suggests that in cases where anti-black people are presented with photographs of black people they concentrate on the common features of this stereotype and ignore those individual characteristics which would be essential for later recognition. Because such a person only notices those features which conform to this pre-existing stereotypic schemata he will be left with the impression that they 'all look alike'. That this is not too fanciful is supported by work carried out by Secord in the 1950s (Secord, Bevan and Katz, 1956). He showed volunteers ten pictures of negroes whose skin colour varied from very light to very dark, and then asked the volunteers to rate these photographs in terms of 'classical' negroid features (e.g. complexion, width of nose). Secord found that his anti-black subjects tended to perceive photographs of blacks as possessing more classic features than did his non-prejudiced subjects. It seems as if Secord's prejudiced volunteers were employing strong visual stereotypes which led them to selectively perceive only those features which conformed to, and confirmed, their stereotype. Other features were given less attention. This perceptual selectivity results in less differentiation and hence greater difficulty in perceiving crucial (identificatory) differences between individual, out-group, faces.

Paradoxically, precisely this conclusion can be drawn from Galper's experiment (1973) (the *one* study which found whites recognized *black* faces better than they did white faces). The white students in this study were markedly pro-black, and indicated this by enrolment in a course of black studies. Note that one would not expect such a finding if white faces were inherently more easy than black faces, but one would expect such findings on the basis of differential familiarity. Galper favours this later suggestion – but the findings are also congruent with the prejudice hypothesis. One suggestive line of British evidence for this third explanation comes from Billig and Milner (1976). They showed that white university students and white working class apprentices had much more difficulty in recognizing black than white faces. In a second study they showed that white police and civilian subjects produced more errors in recognizing black faces than white ones and that differential experience had no appreciable effect on error rates.

It should be noted, however, that this third explanation of a cross-racial effect in person identification (i.e. racial prejudice) is a possible explanation only by a process of elimination in that research suggests that neither the 'inherent difficulty' nor the 'familiarity' hypotheses are appropriate explanations. Further, it is acceptable only if the three possible explanations which we have mentioned are exhaustive, and this is doubtful. Billig and Milner are concerned to point out that their study implies the prejudice argument, but an interpretation in terms of black faces being inherently more difficult to recognize than white faces is similarly not ruled out by the data of their experiment.

In terms of our present concern with possible implications for person recognition, a further group of studies is important for the evidence afforded of possible learning effects on the recognition of out-group faces. Malpass, Lavigueur and Weldon (1973) demonstrated that training in identifying the relevant features of black faces could improve the performance of white subjects to the extent of achieving comparable performance levels on both black and white face recognition. And similarly Elliott, Wills and Goldstein (1973) were able to improve white subjects' recognition of oriental faces by such training. Lavrakas *et al.* (1976) also found that training significantly improved immediate recognition performance (but not long term) by white subjects of black faces. They employed a feature discrimination training task based on concept attainment of 'black face with light eyes' and 'dark eyes and thick lips'. As identikit faces were shown subjects had to respond 'concept' or 'no concept'. When the subject had made five correct responses he or she was asked to say what the concept was. This is a fairly simple training device compared to that of Elliot *et al.* (1973) and Malpass *et al.* (1973) but 'it appears to be as efficient, and more salient' (Lavrakas *et al.*, 1976). While the possibility of training does not here help us in our theory building (all three possible explanations outlined above could account for training effects), it is important in practical terms, especially for the police and people located in high risk areas. In terms of training techniques it would seem to be the case that strategies of scanning and focusing which are beneficial for white faces may not be so for black faces. Ellis (1975) pointed out that white subjects attend to such features as eyes and hair colour, which are less appropriate when applied to black faces, and black subjects concentrate more on face outline and skin colour which, for white faces, may be less discriminating cues than for black faces. For white subjects the most salient feature of a black face is its blackness, which does not, however, convey much discriminating information. Training could 'set' subjects to attend to other features which could prove more useful as discriminating cues, and to forgo the luxury of devoting attention to the most salient but least discriminating feature of a face.

A study which goes some way towards providing a basis for the development of training strategies is one by Ellis, Deregowski and Shepherd (1975). They looked at the frequency with which white and black subjects used different facial features when *describing* faces. While there is no guarantee that faces are encoded verbally, and some evidence that they are not (Goldstein and Chance, 1971; Ellis, 1975), none the less it is a fair assumption, made by Ellis *et al.*, that people will tend to describe those features to which they habitually pay visual attention. Ellis *et al.* clearly demonstrated that whites and blacks use different patterns of reference in the description of faces. These different cultural patterns of attention to facial features are due, according to Ellis, to a learning process whereby strategies are acquired for analysing the classes of faces to which one is most frequently exposed. In the case of white faces details of hair colour and texture, as well as iris colour, prove useful cues for discrimination and the frequent exposure to such faces leads to the effective utilization of these cues for the remembering of white faces but not for black faces. Ellis points out that this argument is not so easily used to explain the differential recognition superiority of black observers of black faces because there is no good reason to suppose that attention to features such as ears, chin, eyebrows, eye and whites of eye, style of hair and face outline would lead to better discrimination by black observers of black compared with white faces in the same way as attention to iris colour and hair texture and colour could prove useful in the discrimination of white but not black faces. The critical difference between the African subjects' response to both black and to white faces is that they mentioned more features of black faces (which could underlie their superior memory for black compared with white faces), whereas the whites, while mentioning an equal number of features, tended for black faces to mention those features which were redundant (e.g. 'dark skin'). This suggests, by extrapolation, that while white subjects deploy their attention widely over black faces their information pick-up is quite redundant, and therefore of little use for later identification. Thus the evidence of white subjects being better for white faces and black subjects being better for black faces could be explained by the fact that white subjects pay attention to highly discriminating features of white faces, which the black subjects ignore, and second, black observers process a greater number of useful or discriminating facial features of black faces than do white subjects, the white subjects tending to focus on redudant features or attributes.

The study by Ellis *et al.* (1975) looked at verbal descriptions (based, presumably, upon visual attentional patterns) of physiognomic characteristics of black and white faces by black and white subjects. A related study which compares Japanese and white faces is one by Goldstein and Chance (1976). This study addressed itself to the basic question of whether white American faces are more heterogeneous and thus more easily discriminated than Japanese faces. That is, whether the variability among structural features of Japanese faces is less than the variability found among facial structures of white Americans. In terms of the findings from a number of studies it seems to be the case that white subjects recognize white faces best, Japanese faces least well and are intermediate for black faces. In terms of explanation, Goldstein and Chance (1976) favour the differential frequency hypothesis and cite as support the study by Elliott *et al.* (1973) where white subject's recognition memory for unfamiliar Japanese faces was significantly improved as a function of training on a task which increased their familiarity with Japanese faces not used in the study. Goldstein and Chance, however, point out that the differential experience hypothesis will not be capable of crucial experimental validation or falsification until it is independently ascertained whether in fact Japanese faces differ in some way from white faces. Goldstein and Chance investigated this latter problem by empirically determining the within-group homogeniety for the two races. If Japanese faces are more alike than white faces then more recognition errors would be expected on Japanese faces irrespective of familiarity with the race as such. Goldstein and Chance therefore hypothesized that if Japanese faces are more alike structurally than white faces then longer inspection times should be observed, and more errors occur, in situations where subjects have to decide whether a pair of Japanese faces are photographs of the same individual or photographs of two different people. Only photographs of males were used. Photographs were projected, in pairs, onto a screen which was situated in front of the subjects. The two photographs could either be of the same person or of two different persons. These researchers found no difference between the time taken to make same or different judgments for Japanese or white faces, and no difference in the number of correct responses for the two types of faces. While the published version of these studies (Goldstein and Chance, 1976) can be faulted methodologically in terms of number and type of photographs used, and number of trials run, the paper presented by Goldstein (1975b) to the Psychology Association corrects a number of these faults and the same results and conclusions emerge, only more strongly.

Goldstein and Chance conclude that these data offer no support for the notion that Japanese faces are more structurally similar, and therefore less discriminable, than white faces. This finding suggests, as Goldstein and Chance point out, that the difference in recognition performance between different races in recognition of other-race faces may reside in storage or retrieval processes rather than the process of recognition. Comparing Ellis *et al.* (1975) and Goldstein and Chance (1976) we have apparently conflicting results. Ellis suggests there are differences in encoding as indexed by verbal description of faces; Goldstein and Chance suggest there is no difference in encoding as suggested by reaction time to make decisions of 'same' or 'different'. The problem with the latter conclusion is that the same objective time to do two different things (responding to white faces and responding to oriental faces) can mask or hide the fact that within this objective similarity vastly different things could be going on, such as differential strategies of perception, encoding and registration. It was a great pity that neither of the two researchers explored a causal relationship by employing the verbal description or decision between 'same' and 'different' as a cover for an unannounced recognition test of the processed photographs. In the absence of this measure the relation of encoding and recognition of black, yellow and white faces by black and white subjects is at best tentative.

MULTI-DIMENSIONAL SCALING AND FACE DIFFERENTIALS

So far we have conducted the discussion into facial memory for white and non-white faces in terms of salient features and their encoding. We argued above that facial features may be a misleading datum and perhaps configurations, patterns and attributes are what should be studied. Research in verbal learning suggest that words have connotative and denotative attributes and that these have important implications for encoding and storage (e.g. Wickens, 1972). One approach to word attribute scaling is the Osgood Semantic Differential (SD) which, when used together with the experimental paradigm of release from pro-active interference (Wickens, 1970), has given valuable evidence on how verbal memory is organized. Could a face differential do the same for visual memory? A start in this direction has been made at Illinois University, in the work of Hurwitz, Wiggins and Jones (1975) and Jones and Hirschberg (1975), and at Aberdeen University some valuable evidence has also been produced (Shepherd, personal communication to first author).

Faces have been used as stimulus objects in such diverse areas of psychology as perception, personality and social interaction (Cohen, 1973; Cross *et al.*, 1971; Hochberg, 1964; Warr and Knapper, 1968), and as a result we know a fair amount about the psychology of faces, e.g. personality traits are readily attributed to facial photographs in a fairly consistent manner (Brunswik, 1956; Secord, 1958; Chapter 3 above) and facial features are readily generated on the basis of verbal, personality-trait, information. Further, faces are readily measurable on a variety of physical and cosmetic variables (Harmon, 1973). These three aspects of the psychology of faces makes possible the generation of a 'psycho-physics of faces' (Hurwitz *et al.*, 1975).

Hurwitz *et al.* have tried to calibrate the personality characteristics or attributes which are salient, relevant and important to facial perception, taking sex and race differences of observers into account. Their facial differential (FD) was constructed along the same lines as Osgood's SD. Basically Hurwitz *et al.* presented photographs of black and white male faces to black and white men and women as asked them to give trait adjectives and phrases describing the likely personality of the person depicted (e.g. pleasant, lively, domineering, etc.). This was made easier by suggesting to the subjects that they should see the situation as if they were describing to a friend a photograph which only they could see. The twenty photographs contained faces which represented variation along major dimensions of facial attributes identified by Wasserman, Wiggins, Jones and Itkin (1974). The adjectives selected by the different subjects were instructive. Women associated pleasant/unpleasant, warm-cold, naive/sophisticated, more often than men. Black subjects associated honest/dishonest, conceited/not conceited, trusting-nontrusting, cool/not cool, more often than white subjects. From this study a set of bipolar adjective scales suggest themselves as relevant and salient for facial attributes. Again, unfortunately, while this study suggests that facial attributes can lead to different personality assessments in the form of verbal labels no relationship with recognition was investigated. Thus what we have so far is that facial attributes can be discerned but unfortunately little data are available from these verbal encoding studies on possible male-female and black-white differences in the recognition of black and white faces. This is an important beginning to the question of encoding dimensions of seen faces, but it is only a beginning. A study which looks more closely at the possibility of multi-dimensional scaling of faces comes from the same stable at Illinois University where Jones and Hirschberg (1975) looked at several dimensions of black and white women's perception of black and white male faces in terms of such things as the structural features and rated attributes of faces; the demographic, personality and attitudinal variables of observers in judgment of faces; and, fundamentally, the basic dimensions of face perception. Female undergraduate students served as subjects. Thirty-two were black and 32 were white, 18 colour transparencies containing front-view face photographs were used as stimuli. There were 9 black and 9 white male photographs. The basic procedure was to project slides in pairs and ask the subjects to judge whether they preferred the left-hand slide, or were indifferent, or preferred the right-hand slide. The subjects were also asked to rate whether the two photographs were very similar or very dissimilar. Over and above these two requirements all subjects rated all displayed photographs on fifteen bipolar adjectives measuring various expressive and attribute characteristics such as intelligent-stupid, threatening-non threatening, mature-immature, dark skinned-light skinned. The conclusions were numerous but for our purposes it was shown that major perceptual dimensions were race, attractiveness, maturity, masculinity, basic shape of face, eyes and a catch-all dimension called gauntness. The important points are that while race of photograph was a highly salient cue most subjects' judgments of similarity were based on several other structural and inferred attributes. At least four other dimensions were crucially involved: maturity, attractiveness, face shape and eye characteristics. Although there were large within and between race differences in the relative salience of these dimensions, it was concluded that, 'the identified dimensions would predict differences in recognition accuracy among faces but with differential contributions for different subjects' (Jones and Hirschberg, 1975).

Now once again we are in command of evidence of individual and group differences in encoding faces and some generalizability and stability is beginning to emerge. What remains to be done is to link these differential encodings to differential performance in recognition scores. The results of the above study suggest some framework for the manipulation and control of relevant stimulus and individual difference variables in our quest for a greater understanding of the psychology of person identification and recognition. The one nagging doubt in our minds is that, like factor analysis in general, you only get out what you put in (e.g. Butcher, 1968) and what we are getting are statistical or logical factors, not psychological factors. However, if we find that labelling of faces aids recognition then this pessimistic view could be dispelled, and this is precisely what we will find in the studies by McKelvie (1976b) and Chance and Goldstein (1976) discussed in Chapter 6.

JUST HOW GOOD CAN FACIAL IDENTIFICATION BE?

So far then we have looked at the perceptual, encoding end of face perception and memory, but what of the retrieval end and the psychological factors which affect this. To begin to answer this question of just how good facial identification can be we go back to the data cited earlier which shows correct identification of face photographs is about 80 per cent. This figure has emerged from our review of relevant studies which have supplied sufficient information. In terms of white faces and immediate recognition performance, the percentage of correct recognition has varied from 96 per cent to 54 per cent with, as we have said, the average being about 79 per cent (Cross *et al.*, 1971; Ellis *et al.*, 1973; Goldstein and Chance, 1974; Hochberg and Galper, 1967; Malpass and Kravitz, 1969; Scapinello and Yarmey, 1970; Shepherd and Ellis, 1973; Yin, 1969). In terms of white faces and delay in testing Shepherd and Ellis (1973) showed decreases from 87 per cent correct identification after viewing immediately to 80 per cent at six days and 71 per cent at thirty-five days delay. Shepherd *et al.* (1974) found correct recognition to be 71 per cent after twenty-four hours delay, and Goldstein and Chance found no difference between identification accuracy at no delay and forty-eight hours delay. Most of these studies have informed subjects of later recognition tests but some have not, and it seems to make little difference (e.g. Bower and Karlin (1974) still got hit rates of 80 per cent when faces had merely been rated for 'likeableness' or 'honesty', and their subjects had not been told of a later recognition task). However, and this is the point, these base-line hit rates need to be qualified in so many ways that they should not be employed to support the case for sound eyewitness testimony. Such qualifications have been implicit in much of what we have said above.

In the light of these qualifications Goldstein (in press) has this to say:

> The variety and scope of the evidence implicating the *general* unreliability of eye witness testimony is so well documented that it would almost be impossible to find a psychologist (or for that matter a sociologist or psychiatrist) who did not believe that most eyewitnesses are untrust-worthy reporters of what happened, how it happened, and to whom it happened.

How can this be explained? The reasons are numerous: Clifford (1975) suggested that, 'Laboratory studies create unreality by using overlong exposure durations, non-aroused subjects and isomorphic relationships between situations of viewing and situations of recognition.' Over and above these problems there is the question of whether research with photographs is legitimate evidence for an understanding of real-life recognition of faces.

Our everyday memory for faces is good, but this type of memory differs in several important respects from an eyewitness's memory for faces. Our everyday recognition of people is based on either multiple exposures or long single exposures. Laboratory studies have used single exposures stretching from 1 to 30 seconds. Crime episodes on the other hand may produce perceptions of faces which involve single exposures of short durations, whilst the face is dynamic and not static. Can we really equate a memory for a face seen once with a memory for a face seen many times? The jury may extrapolate inappropriately from our 'taken for granted' good memory for faces seen repeatedly or for long exposures, to memory for faces seen once, momentarily, and possibly, under poor perceptual conditions. This extrapolation is doubly doubtful because we traditionally see familiar faces in familiar places – witness the case where you walk past a friend in unfamiliar surroundings without recognizing him, or you cannot place him for a few minutes. This is because the context has changed and thus one crutch of our everyday, good, person recognition has disappeared and our memory for faces is shown to be drastically reduced. How much more is this the case when we are investigating an eyewitness's recognition of a seen criminal? Simulation studies suggest that context effects are crucial and laboratory studies show them to be clearly relevant. Context is important in two senses. First, by reconstructing the crime or situation of viewing, the context can cue the witness's memory of what took place. Second, in identification cases one does not merely have to identify the subject but rather one must identify the suspect as the person who was perceived in the original criminal context, and these are not the same thing. Brown, Deffenbacher and Sturgill (1977) looked at this very problem. They point out that, 'although recognition memory for scenes and faces has been shown to be generally quite good, it should not be supposed that memory for the circumstances of their encounter is at all comparable.' The context cuing effect, where memory is shown to be better if learning and memory take place in the same place, has been known for a long time (e.g. Abernethy, 1940). In one of the studies quoted in Chapter 2 (Standing, Conezio and Haber, 1970) memory for pictures was observed to be extremely good. Here subjects were shown pictures varying in orientation and then, after different retention intervals, were asked to identify which of a pair of pictures had been seen before, and its previous orientation. While subjects were able to recognize the pictures as old (seen before) with high accuracy, their ability to recall whether it was in the same or different orientation was greatly reduced at long delay between initial perception and eventual recognition, compared with short delay. This could represent the fading away of non-important surface structure but the retention of deep structure as mentioned above. This initial perception of surface structure and simultaneous generation of deep structure, then the storage of deep structure and loss of surface structure, and then the eventual 'recognition' of both surface structure and deep structure has vital implications for eyewitness testimony. It involves the possibility of prefabrication or unconscious transfer. Prefabrication and unconscious transfer will be discussed elsewhere, but for the moment we will look at the fact that in criminal identification we are asking the eyewitness to do two things: first, to identify a seen face, and second, to place that face in the criminal situation. A real-life case was quoted in Chapter 2, where this conceptual distinction was shown to be a reality: the witness correctly identified the suspect as familiar but he wrongly placed him at the scene of the crime. Laboratory studies show this type of breakdown to be a readily replicable fact. Brown *et al.* (1977), in their first study, presented subjects with twenty-five pictures of faces in one room, and two hours later in another, radically different room, presented twenty-five more such pictures. Two days later they showed subjects 100 pictures of faces, in pairs, with one of each pair having been previously presented and the other a new face. The subjects were asked to indicate for each pair the picture previously seen, and the room in which it had been presented. This should not have been as difficult as it sounds because subjects had been warned before they saw the pictures for the first time that they would be asked to recall both whether they had seen the photograph before and in which room it had been shown. Recognition was 96 per cent correct, but specification of the viewing room was only 56 per cent correct, chance being 50 per cent. This artificial laboratory experiment could thus have predicted the real-life case quoted by Professor Houts where a witness correctly recognized a face but located it wrongly. More specifically, a witness called to identify a suspect could have had one or more of six types of visual experience of that suspect. The witness could have seen the suspect at the crime, seen him in police photo albums, seen him in the album and line-up, seen the suspect in the newspapers after he (the witness) had observed the crime, and perhaps also identified him from photographs and line-ups, seen him at other times and in other places, or not have seen him at all. It is rather obvious that if a witness is called to identify a person in a line-up his identification could be a function of seeing or not seeing him in any of the possible combinations of the above. In Brown *et al.*'s second study witnesses were told that they were going to see two groups of five people whom they were to inspect closely for twenty-five seconds. They were also told that they would be asked to pick these people out from photo spreads later that evening and from a line-up the following week. The two groups of five persons were the 'criminals'. (Some of these criminals had 'mugshots' taken some did not.) One-and-a-half hours later fifteen mugshots were shown. These fifteen photographs included five of the criminals, five people who would be seen in the line-up one week hence, and five non-criminal and non-line-up persons. The witnesses were asked to indicate for each mugshot whether or not that person had been seen earlier in front of the class and then give a confidence rating for their answer. One week later four line-ups were staged. These line-ups comprised all possible amounts and kinds of prior visual experience on the part of the witness in the sense that the line-up members could have been seen as a criminal, seen as a criminal and in mugshots, only as a mugshot, or seen neither in mugshot nor as a criminal. The witnesses were asked whether or not each person in the line-up had been standing in front of the class the previous week, and whether the person's mugshot had been shown, and to give their confidence for each answer. In the first identification phase (recognizing criminals from mugshots) one and one half hours after perception, correct recognition was approximately 72 per cent, false identification was 45 per cent and confidence ratings were unrelated to accuracy. At the one week delay line-up a number of questions were asked, the first of which was whether the persons in the line-up had also appeared in the mugshots. Forty-seven per cent of criminals who had not been present in mugshots were so indicated. Twenty per cent of the line-up persons who were neither seen as criminals nor in mugshots were said to have appeared in mugshots one week earlier.

The most important question asked was whether the persons on the line-up had been seen as a criminal. Criminals were correctly selected 65 per cent of the time. Criminals without mugshots were correctly selected 51 per cent of the time, while those who appeared on mugshots but were not criminals were selected as criminals 20 per cent of the time, and those on the line-up seen for the first time were selected as criminals on 8 per cent of occasions. Thus there is one chance in five that a mugshot viewing could cause wrongful identification of a person as a seen criminal, and one chance in twelve of an innocent person being so accused.

These rates of false accusation were achieved under conditions of minimum biasing of either the mugshots or the line-up, and under very long initial exposure durations (twenty-five seconds). Under biased conditions or with real-life short exposures many more false accusations would occur, as suggested by Buckhout and as discussed in Chapter 2.

Goldstein's statement is less of a paradox also when we consider real-life targets. We have argued and shown earlier that real-life situations cause marked decrement in identification accuracy but one study by Laughery, cited in Goldstein (in press), reports 84 per cent correct recognition of a single live target when subjects looked for a photograph of this person in a group of 148 distractors. It ought to be pointed out, however, that the target person was exposed for thirty seconds! Laughery reports a second study where the target was either a black or a white person. Recognition memory for the black target by white subjects was 55 per cent correct. The white target was correctly identified 96 per cent of the time. In a related experiment Alexander (Goldstein, in press) investigated recognition memory for one target person, but during the study session subjects were shown four colour photographs depicting various poses of the target face for a total of thirty seconds. Performance was measured with one target and 149 distractor slides. Overall recognition accuracy was 55 per cent. The recognition accuracy quoted under simulated crime episodes in Chapter 2 clearly produces evidence of much poorer performance than this.

A consideration of false positives is the last factor we shall examine in attempting to resolve Goldstein's apparently paradoxical statement. Most studies have given little consideration to false positives, that is the false identification of a person or his photograph as the target when in fact he is not. This has crucial implications for line-up and mugshot procedures, but is seldom discussed. The studies quoted earlier by Buckhout where he looked at impeachment by subjects in blank line-ups is crucial evidence. Goldstein (in press) quotes an unpublished study in which he presented observers with three live targets for either five or thirty seconds duration, and then later asked them to select the targets from either a five picture line-up, or a five man line-up. The thirty-second exposure observers were correct in 100 per cent of cases with line-ups after fifteen days and 90 per cent of the time with photographs after fifteen days. This is incredible memory for faces even allowing for the unrealistic exposure durations, but it became much less impressive when false positives are taken into account; 44 per cent of the subjects impeached themselves. As Goldstein puts it, 'additional information about false recognition will only make the case against eyewitnesses testimony even stronger.'

So far then in this chapter we have looked at how good or bad memory is for a seen person as measured by recognition, that is the witness merely had to express a feeling of familiarity concerning the target. As we argued in Chapter 2 recognition tends to give the highest estimate of how good memory can be, and depending on whether we consider memory for pictures or for real-life, in the flesh, targets, the estimate of witness reliability varies markedly; from about 80 per cent to about 30 per cent. In the conduct of law enforcement the police do use recognition as a means of utilizing witness memory (e.g. by the use of identification parades and photo albums), but they also use methods of recall and cued recall, and it is to these we now wish to turn our attention. On sound theoretical grounds one would predict that recall would give low estimates of memory capacity, with cued recall giving intermediate estimates relative to recall and recognition. To recap on what was said in Chapter 2, when the police have no suspect to be recognized, and an album search has failed they have no option but to institute recall and cued recall procedures. These procedures are predominantly the photo-fit, the identikit or the use of artist's impressions. These all initially involve recall on the part of the subject, but then eventually cued recall occurs because the witness can qualify his assertions ('he had a sharper chin') in the light of what the officer either selects or produces, and further a visual representation can help 'jog' (cue) the witness's memory. The remainder of this chapter will assess the use and efficacy of these police recall techniques.

METHOD OF FACE RECALL: PHOTO-FIT AND ARTIST'S SKETCHES

At present there are three different photo-fit kits for constructing faces of male caucasians, male Afro-Asians and female caucasians. Each kit is made up of a large number of alternative and separate photographs of five facial features (eyes, mouth, nose, chin and forehead/hair) and those desiring to construct a face pick out the parts which best resemble the face they are trying to reconstruct. (Accessories such as glasses or a beard can also be added.) This system was devised by Jacques Penry and was first employed in Britain in 1969. It replaced the similar identikit system which simply used line drawings of various parts of the faces. Soon after the introduction of the photo-fit technique a survey of its use was undertaken by the Police Scientific Development Branch and it was noted that the kit was often used with some measure of satisfaction (King, 1971), and a number of real-life successes due to its employment have been reported. In a more recent survey conducted by the Home Office (Darnbrough, 1977) it was found that in 1975 on average eighty-four photo-fits were constructed per police force. Some forces reported on the time lapse between an incident and a related photo-fit being constructed. This was less than twenty-four hours in 13 per cent of cases and was between twenty-four and forty-eight hours in 20 per cent of the cases. Twenty-nine per cent involved a delay of between two and five days and the remaining 36 per cent being made up six days or more after the incident. Eight per cent of the photo-fits related to homicide, attempted murder or grievous bodily harm; 13 per cent to rape or other sexual offences; 68 per cent to robbery, theft or burglary; and 11 per cent to other types of incident. When asked to indicate how useful photo-fits had been in each case in which they were used in a six month period the relevant investigating police officers said that for crimes which had been cleared up photo-fit was 'entirely responsible' in 5 per cent of cases, 'very useful' in 17 per cent, 'useful' in 33 per cent, 'not very useful' in 20 per cent, and 'of no use at all' in 25 per cent. Concerning the actual construction of the 1,090 photo-fits, before each was constructed 1,077 witnesses had given a verbal description of the suspect to the investigating officer whereas 13 had not. The order of selection of the features which make up a face was decided by the witness in 7.5 per cent of cases and by the operator helping the witness to construct the photo-fit in 92.5 per cent of cases. The actual order in which the photo-fits were built up tended to be first the forehead, then the chin, then the eyes, followed by the nose and then the mouth, with facial hair, spectacles and other accessories being added at the end. This order applied both when the witness or the photo-fit operator was in charge of the order of feature selection. We have discussed experiments which suggest that the eyes and mouth are important for identification, so it is worth noting here that the eyes were the first facial attribute chosen to make up the photo-fit in less than 2 per cent of cases (though they were the second attribute chosen in 26 per cent of cases) and that the mouth was chosen first in 1 per cent of cases and second in less than 2 per cent. This suggests that while we may spend most of our time looking at the eyes and mouth this may be in order to gather information about mood, and to communicate, and thus little encoding for memory of these features may go on. However, before we can accept this line of reasoning we would have to ensure that construction-order is not an artifact of both the set-up of the photo-fit kit itself, and the fact that the construction of the photo-fit is operator-guided in the vast proportion of cases.

Those features which were changed three or more times once an initial selection had been made were the eyes in 24 per cent of all cases, the nose in 18 per cent, the mouth in 17 per cent, the chin in 15 per cent and the forehead in 8 per cent, there being 18 per cent of cases in which none of the features was changed three or more times. When asked, 'How easy is it to select a more suitable part from the kit when the witness describes what is wrong with his first choice?' seven per cent of operators said that it was 'easy', 60 per cent 'fairly easy', 28 per cent 'quite difficult', 4.5 per cent 'difficult' and 0.5 per cent 'very difficult'. In 61 per cent of cases freehand additions to the final photo-fits were needed and on 39 per cent of occasions they were not, this giving some indication of the adequacy of the raw photo-fit. When asked, 'Did it prove possible to make a photo-fit that was acceptable to the witness?' the photo-fit operators indicated that on 94 per cent of occasions this was the case. The average time taken for a photo-fit to be made up was forty-five minutes, with a range from fifteen minutes to three hours.

This survey is by far the most informative that has been undertaken concerning the use of photo-fit and its findings are of importance since the sample size was large and inclusive. From the survey it would seem that a number of very interesting questions arise which would be amenable to experimental analysis. However, the actual number of direct investigations of the photo-fit by psychologists is woefully small.

Perhaps the only experimental study which directly sets out to test photo-fit is that of Ellis, Shepherd and Davies (1975). Here it was found that, 'even when allowed a continuous view of a face made up of photo-fit features subjects were unable to reconstruct it perfectly using the kit', and that, 'when reconstructing from memory, performance was substantially poorer'. In this study each reconstructed face could receive a maximum score of five points if each of the five photo-fit features had been correctly selected. The average score when subjects were reconstructing with the face present was two out of five and when reconstructing from memory the score fell to one out of five. However, in this paper the authors provide no information concerning how similar to the original face were the attributes that were incorrectly selected. Since the photo-fit kit provides a great many possibilities (roughly 100) for each of the five features such data is very necessary. A reconstruction could have selected the 'wrong' nose but since there were a great many noses to choose from, the 'wrong' one could have closely resembled the original one but have been deemed an error. Though the findings of Ellis *et al.* are of interest they fail to provide any information on how much worse witnesses might be at providing information about an individual if photo-fit were not available, and this of course, is the crucial question. These authors' second experiment has more ecological validity. Here good and poor reconstructors from the first experiment made up photo-fits of facial photographs. These photographs were then shown one at a time to seventy-two other observers who had to pick the face which matched the photo-fit from an array of thirty-six facial photographs. In this more meaningful situation correct identifications occurred with greater frequency than could be expected by chance, with the photo-fits of the good reconstructors leading to more correct selections than those of the poor reconstructors, but it was concluded that 'the results leave room for improvement' since on many occasions the wrong face was picked out as being the original source for the assembled photo-fit.

While the Ellis *et al.* (1975) study is the only published report on photo-fit this research team has recently completed a large project into many other aspects of the psychology of photo-fit construction, and have kindly made their results available to us (Ellis, Davies (with Shepherd); 'An investigation of the photo-fit system for recalling faces', Report to the SSRC), a summary of which appears below.

Subjects spent most of their time selecting the upper part of the face, especially brow and hair line, relative to the lower parts such as mouth and chin. This could be due either to the fact that in the kit the number of upper head features outnumber the lower face features, or because most attention is deployed to the upper face and head during initial perception of a face and thus the constructor has more information available about this part of the face and hence has more precise criteria as to just what is acceptable as a 'resemblance'. One other possibility could be that in the experience of Ellis *et al.*, police operators begin at the top of the head and work down, and thus the greater time spent on this part of the face by the subjects could simply represent unfamiliarity with the task. This observation by Ellis could also explain the ambiguity we noted in the Home Office finding that the actual order in which a photo-fit was built up was forehead first, contrary to what would be predicted from facial feature fixations. The fact was that 92.5 per cent of all constructions in the Home Office report were officer-directed. Ellis *et al.* felt that the large number of features in the kit interfered with accurate reconstruction, and initially most constructors felt dissatisfied with their completed effort. However, after modification 75 per cent were reasonably satisfied. It was found that there was little difference between constructions generated under experienced and non-experienced operators.

Most interesting of all, however, were the negative findings. In terms of delay it seemed to make no difference to the accuracy of construction whether the construction took place immediately, two days, seven days or twenty-three days later. Also it seemed to make no difference whether the person had observed the target for long or short durations, or had been told to remember him or not. Most surprisingly it also made no difference whether the face was present or not while construction was going on. In terms of possible screening by police of witnesses for accuracy and reliability it is unfortunate that this research team found that photo-fit construction was not correlated with sex, imagery ability, personality type (field-dependence/independence), or objectively assessed recognition accuracy of the observers. Usefully, however, Ellis *et al.* found that constructing a photo-fit did not interfere with (render poorer) eventual recognition of the target person. Previous research would have suggested that asking people to recall faces would reduce later recognition performance (Belbin, 1950; Kay and Skemp, 1956). This is important for law enforcement.

Equally important for law enforcement development was the finding that one race finds it difficult to construct a photo-fit of a face from another race. Photo-fits of well-known faces were rated as fairly good resemblances (of Heath, Wilson and Thorpe), thus suggesting, in opposition to one of their earlier findings, that very frequent or long exposure may have the effect of increasing the accuracy of photo-fit construction.

In line with one of the main arguments of this book it was interesting to find that attitudes and stereotypes can materially affect photo-fit construction of a seen face. Housewives acted as subjects in one study, and were all shown the same face. However, for half the subjects they were led to believe that they were seeing the face of a murderer, while the other half of the subjects were led to believe they were looking at a life-boat captain. The photo was then removed and the women were asked to construct a photo-fit of the face they had seen. After completing this task they were asked to rate the target face on a number of bipolar adjectives such as pleasant-unpleasant, intelligent-non intelligent. The two groups differed on eight of the nine scales (the one scale showing no difference being 'hard-soft'). The next stage of the experiment involved presenting the constructed photo-fit faces to a new group of subjects who had to rate these two faces on the same bipolar adjectives. The 'life-boat photo-fit' was rated as significantly more attractive and intelligent than the 'murder photo-fit'. This strongly argues (as we have done) that the nature of the crime 'witnessed' can seriously distort the witness's memory for the criminal.

The overall impression from this research is, however, essentially negative concerning the efficacy of the photo-fit. Many of the findings of Ellis *et al.* are clouded by 'floor effects' due to the fact that the kit 'is not a sensitive enough instrument to allow people adequately to represent their memory for a face'. The basic finding in the vast majority of their experiments was that photo-fit constructions were characterized by poor likeness.

Stemming from their research findings Ellis *et al.* suggest certain improvements in eliciting face recall by the photo-fit. They suggest that the division of facial features into only five parts is too crude, more divisions are required. Allied to this they suggest that a greater number of separate features should be available for upper head areas, but they are aware that such an increase could serve to confuse the witness. They also suggest the opposite to increasing single features, viz. the development of prototype kits. This tentative suggestion comes from the finding that many of the subjects began construction by stating that the target person looked like some famous personality. By fragmenting the image, or face gestalt, that witnesses may have of the seen criminal, the photo-fit may actually be working against good recall. This face prototype kit may require expert police artists, or a computer-graphics system, which is in fact being developed at Cambridge University. At the moment there are other possible explanations of the photo-fit's weakness.

A number of psychological studies have been conducted which

have some bearing on photo-fit though the authors of these works do not mention the implications that their results have for this technique. Gilbert and Bakan (1973), McCurdy (1949), Wolff (1945), Lindzey, Prince and Wright (1952) and Coltheart (1975) all found that one half-side of an individual's face can be noticeably different from the other half, a fact which photo-fit and other recognition aids should, but as yet do not, take into account even though Ellis (1975) believes that these asymmetries do not matter very much. Wolff (1933) noted, as did Gilbert and Bakan, that individuals were more likely to recognize themselves if shown a composite of two left halves of their own face than if shown two right halves (left being from an observer's point of view). Wolff also noted that people are poor at recognizing their own profile photographs, but this finding should be compared with that by Laughery, Alexander and Lane (1971) who found pose position made no difference to recognition accuracy. In the study of Fisher and Cox discussed above it was found that when they progressively revealed photographs of famous people laterally, left-sided features (to the observer) aided recognition twice as much as did similar right-sided ones.

Another problem with photo-fit is its inability to portray expression. While Ellis (1975) concluded that, 'there is no evidence to suggest that the expression of a face has much bearing on the memory processes underlying facial recognition', Galper (1970) believes that, 'no face is expressionless' and that, 'the perception of expression is an integral part of the viewing of a face'. Both may be correct because the crucial problem with expression is that it can change between the initial situation of viewing and the eventual situation of recalling or recognizing. This is less of a problem for identification parades, because the participants can be asked to smile, stare, etc., but it is a real problem for photo-fit construction. One can suggest how expression may mislead mechanized face recognizers which rely on inter-feature measurements but there exist few studies which have rigorously examined the role of expression in the human recognition of faces. Sorce and Campos (1974) found 'that facial expression is an important parameter of facial recognition', and their results could be taken as support for the contention that the greater the difference between a face's expression on initial viewing and on later recognition testing the poorer is recognition performance. Thus Ellis's (1975) statement would seem to be in need of reformulation especially since, as discussed in Chapter 3, facial expression can play a major role in the operation of applying stereotypes. The photo-fit system also lacks the ability to portray a representative range of facial expression. Its origin-·ator, Penry (1971), acknowledges to some extent the role of expression in determining the exact visual input that an observer of a face will receive. However, his suggested range of shapes for the five facial features is a function more of the differences between various faces when each is expressionless than it is of the range of shapes that a single person's facial features can adopt (especially the eyes and mouth). This lack of expression is one reason why many people find the photo-fit faces circulated by the police rather strange, even eerie.

We consider that facial expression can play a major role in recognition especially since witnesses frequently fail to notice facial features like eye colour, type of nose, beard, etc., and instead they talk about people being fierce looking, having staring eyes or hard mouths (Clifford, 1975). Warr and Knapper (1968) suggest that witnesses' descriptions are likely to be in terms of the emotional impressions they gained of the individual rather than in terms of his anatomy and clothing (e.g. the witness may be able to say only that the assailant 'looked menacing'). It is certainly true that the subjective, emotional impressions one gains from perceiving individuals are the important things for interactional purposes.

One might ask if any other method of arriving at a pictorial representation of a face would have greater success. A similar method to photo-fit involves an artist attempting to draw a face based upon information provided by a witness. This procedure is used widely in the USA and sometimes in Britain too. Few experiments have examined this method but one by Harmon and Murray-Hill (1971) used two trained and practised artists from a US law enforcement agency. Three of six photographs of separate individuals were given to each artist who was required to compile a written description of each photograph. The descriptions were given to the other artist who then attempted to draw likenesses based on the descriptions. The resulting drawings were shown to thirty persons who had 'all seen the suspects often'. Only thirteen of these thirty observers correctly recognized the portrayed individuals and five of these were individuals who recognized themselves. However, when the artists drew the faces in the presence of the photographs recognition performance rose to 90 per cent. Amongst other things this study highlights a problem which was discussed in Chapter 2, namely that of translating from verbal to pictorial information and vice versa.

Penry (1971) notes that a witness may describe someone as having 'a sensual mouth' and that the police would re-phrase this into 'full-lipped'. Such re-phrasing, the non-utilization of more impressionistic data, seems inappropriate. It is even possible that 'a sensual mouth' may be a more widely understood and discriminating part of a description than something seemingly less subjective (e.g. 'dark complexion'). Begg (1971) notes that memory storage of information is not in the form of the physical stimuli initially perceived but is in the form of the meaning the perceiver gives to such stimuli. Few, if any, studies have been conducted to see to what extent the words presently used by the police in descriptions are understood and can be accurately employed by the general public.

One way to cut out this visual-verbal loop would be to have the witness do his own drawing of the seen face. In the unpublished research quoted above by Ellis *et al.* they did just this. They found that sketches made in the presence of a face were actually quite good, and were significantly better than photo-fits constructed to the same face under the same conditions. This strongly suggests that if the general public could be educated in basic drawing skills then police information concerning seen criminals could be greatly improved.

MAN-MACHINE INTERACTIONS

Another method of arriving at a pictorial likeness of a seen person as a function of a witness's recollections is to have the witness interacting with some sort of machine which rapidly provides possible faces for the witness to manipulate.

In Chapter 6 we shall refer to the influence of the style of questioning upon recollection. Questioning strategy is one of the factors which has been examined by investigations of man-machine systems of human recognition. Some of the procedures which have been developed have tried to avoid relying exclusively upon witnesses' verbal recall (the problems of which were already discussed in Chapter 2). Photo-fit is a procedure which is capable of being used in this way. Other more complex approaches are available.

Goldstein and Harmon have published details of some of their studies and it is probable that other investigations have been performed in this area but have remained unpublished for security or commercial reasons. Sakai, Nagao and Kanade (1972) presented pictorial stimuli to their computer which measured various facial dimensions. Their fully automated system was fairly good at recognizing most faces (552 correct out of 607 trials) but it was completely flummoxed by faces with either a beard or glasses. Human perceivers are also likely to suffer from the illusions that some facial accessories may, by design, create (e.g. a man with a pointed chin can be advised to grow a concealing beard). Sakai *et al.* concluded that a successful mechanized system would need to be extremely complex with a combination of linear and hierarchical searches and many sub-routines.

Goldstein and Harmon's studies have employed man-machine interactions. They have found (Harmon, 1973) that the most efficient recognition system is one in which a human observer first of all informs the computer of the nature of any outstanding stimulus features and then the computer asks the human observer to provide it with information about other features which it selects to be the next most useful. They claimed that most human observers could accurately and promptly inform the computer (using five-point rating scales) of the nature of various facial attributes. 'Trained observers were in excellent agreement with the official [i.e. measured] feature values' (Goldstein *et al.*, 1972). They did find that some observers were better at this task than others and that, 'one subject was consistently poor'.

In one study (Goldstein, Harmon and Lesk, 1971) ten trained observers each rated 256 portrait photographs of middle-aged, white males for each of 34 physical attributes on five-point scales. The authors concluded that, 'performance across raters was reasonably reliable.' However, for more than half of the photographs there was at least one attribute for which the observers' ratings were spread across three or more points on the five-point scale. In their later studies these authors removed from the rating task those attributes for which in 1971 there was substantial inter-observer disagreement, or which did not discriminate between faces. Thus 22 features (of the original 34) remained on the rating list. Further photographs were rated for these attributes in the above manner and given such information about a photograph the computer can come up with the photograph in its memory bank which has the best 'goodness of fit' to the information supplied by the human.

Harmon (1973) found that the quickest way for such a system to work is not for the human to go through the attribute list in any totally pre-prescribed order but for him to select those features of the face which he believes to be outstanding and to straightaway inform the computer of these. If the computer then requires further information, it will ask for details of those features which it knows will discriminate quickest between the memory subset it has selected on the basis of the information supplied by the human observer. Goldstein, Harmon and Lesk (1972) noted that, 'Humans are almost perfect at selecting the features that are the most discriminating for any one photograph.' With this system the target group was reduced to 4 per cent of the total number of faces in the computer memory on 99 per cent of trials.

Goldstein and Harmon believe that a system employing human observer plus computer is more efficient than employing either alone. They found that when faced with an array of photographs and given verbal information about the target face one attribute at a time human observers are only correct on about 50 per cent of trials when employing the strategy of retaining all the photographs they believe to possess the announced attributes until only one face remains. The authors concluded that, 'such a binary selection is too rigid' because the observers often discarded the true target face too early in their search. It is likely that a system such as that of Goldstein and Harmon which does not employ strict binary selection or rejection (by virtue of its weighting of the discriminability of various features and by its subsequent computations of 'goodness of fit') would be superior to the binary and serial processing system which might be employed by humans (as suggested by Bradshaw and Wallace, 1971). Furthermore, humans are very poor at utilizing negative information (Bourne, 1966).

Serial processing often relies upon prolonged linear searches which are not conducive to good performance in humans. Laughery *et al.* (1974) found that recognition performance was an inverse function of the position in the search list of the target face. Such a finding (plus the related work of Anderson (1965) on impression formation) is likely to have important implications for present practices. Laughery suggests that a more fruitful procedure would consist of some 'hierarchical zeroing-in process'. Goldstein and Harmon's system appears to meet this requirement and is a promising development in the area of person recognition. However, a major problem for any mechanized person-recognizer are the changes in the size and inter-distance of many facial features which are brought about by changes in facial expression. If it is true that the CIA are supporting the development of a scanner which examines the profile outline of a face, compares it with computer memory and then decides whether the person who has, for example, just walked along the narrow gangway near passport control, is a threat, then all a thinking terrorist needs to do is to 'pull a face' or blow his nose for this system to be baffled.

Such mechanized systems have been developed to aid recognition of particular stimuli; that is to select from an array that stimulus which is most like the one initially perceived. What few, if any, of them are yet able to do is to perceive something, to store this information, and then to produce it unaided upon request. A video system can do this but it needs to be in the appropriate place at the right time. Human beings are quite good at such recall, they can remember and retrieve things without the aid of the cues present in recognition tasks. However, what human being are prone to do and what machines are unlikely to do is to permit their expectancies and stereotypes to play a role.

5 Identification by visual, non-facial cues and by voice

It is common knowledge that often we can recognize others by their faces but we may ask if any other visual aspects of individuals aid our recognition of them. The questions asked by police of witnesses suggests that there are. Details of age, height and body-build are frequently sought and we might add to these a number of more dynamic, but as yet neglected, aspects such as the way people walk, the gestures they make and the way they dress. As Supt Allen (1950) suggested, 'It is the many little things such as body-build, walk, deportment and mannerisms that we should study.' It is also likely that we can recognize people by the way they speak.

BODY MOVEMENT

Person recognition via visual, non-facial cues is a topic which has largely been ignored by psychologists. One reason for this is the difficulty of describing many of these cues in words. Body movement, for example, is a cue which falls into this category. It is an unfortunate fact that few rigorous studies have been conducted in this area and this has led Warr and Knapper (1968) to state that, 'Variables like style of walking, footsteps, hand movements and mannerisms are all inputs which may warrant more serious investigation.' These and similar variables may not prove to be as discriminating as facial ones but they cannot fail to aid recognition especially in situations such as cross-racial perception, in which facial discrimination is often poor.

In most cases of identification the witness will have seen the suspect move. Eisenberg (1937) stated that,

> The expressive movement of an individual is his style of behaviour and this is relatively independent of the particular situation. Thus we all recognize our friends by the way they walk, talk, eat, sneeze, move their hands, write, dress, dance, sit in a chair, and so on. The question then is, does the individual perform all these various expressive movements in somewhat the same way?

The study of person recognition by visual, non-facial cues seems worthwhile, especially since these factors are frequently not under the conscious, voluntary control of the person being perceived – a point noted by Allport (1937), Ekman and Friesen (1969) and Allen (1950), who provides an interesting example of a murderer being apprehended through the recognition of his gait.

Walking is perhaps the largest human movement that one can commonly observe and thus it is likely to have a number of parameters which could play a role in recognition. Home Office Circular no. 9/1969 on identification parades states that, 'Sometimes there may be something peculiar in the suspect's gait and if the witness decides to see the person walk there is no objection to this.' The problem caused by the lack of an adequate descriptive vocabulary applies here and as Morton and Fuller (1952) noted, 'The multiplicity of the mobile parts and the simultaneous actions of many joints give human locomotion the complexity of detail that defies analysis.' Kreezer and Glanville (1937) listed what they believed to be a number of quantifiable aspects of gait (such as relation of feet to ground, movements of legs, movements of arms, position of head, position of trunk, grace, rhythm and defects), but their method of analysis requires the filming of individuals and subsequent single-frame examination. Such a procedure may be useful in some circumstances but it seems inappropriate to eyewitness situations. However, Kreezer and Glanville did make the point that verbal description of gait is extremely difficult whereas its visual recognition might not be. Allport and Vernon (1933) noted that the psychological dilemma facing investigators in this area concerns the problem of either (i) following a statistical-mechanical procedure which yields crude successions of single elements which never give a living picture (Prost, 1965; Zug, 1972), or (ii) having a more intuitive approach which retains vitality but which is difficult to quantify and communicate.

The only study found by the authors to examine directly person recognition by gait cues was conducted by Wolff (1933). Here, unknown to the individuals concerned, the gaits of a number of acquainted and like-dressed persons were filmed in a standard setting. It was found that the subjects were unable to recognize their friends or wives solely by watching the films but they could sometimes recognize themselves even though they may never have seen themselves on film before. A few studies have examined how consistent individuals are in their gait patterns, a necessary pre-requisite for identification. Borg, Edgren and Markland (1973) noted reliable individual differences in preferred walking speed on two occasions one month apart, and Allport and Vernon (1933) noted high across-session reliabilities in walking speed and stride-length.

Other bodily movements have been studied. Jones and Hanson (1961, 1962) filmed the movement of a fluorescent light source attached to individuals' heads whilst they rose from a sitting to a standing position. It was found that the resultant 'movement profiles are highly characteristic for individual subjects' who either performed the task eight times during a single session or returned fifteen months later. Frey and von Cranach (1973) observed the body movement variability of a number of individuals during six separate mealtimes. They found that the inter-individual variability was much greater than the intra-individual variability with hand movement showing the greatest reliability. (Annett (1970) notes that handedness is a fairly stable human characteristic and suggests that manual speed may also be so, as does Eisenberg (1937).) Similar findings were noted for dyadic interactions. Frey and von Cranach concluded, that 'The results of these studies therefore permit the conclusion that individual characteristics of variability in body movement remain fairly stable under changing conditions.' Thus, there is some evidence over and above Eisenberg and Reichline's (1939) own limited findings for their belief that, 'We know (i) that people vary markedly in their expressive movements; (ii) that expressive movements are fairly stable characteristics of the organism; (iii) that expressive movements are interrelated within a given organism.'

The validity of this last point receives support from studies by both Bruchon (1969) and Wolff (1933), the latter author noting that observers' descriptions of what they expected individuals' personalities to be like, having seen a film of them (from the waist down) walking along, closely matched personality estimates of the same individuals gained two years earlier from their handwriting and speech. Similarly, Allport and Vernon (1933) noted that the various expressive movements of an individual are to some extent interrelated. However, they noted that speed of walking did not correlate at all highly with other measures of speed (e.g. reading, finger tapping, counting) and they concluded that, 'There is no conclusive evidence for a single pervasive "personal tempo".' Instead their 'results favour the postulating of three speed factors – verbal, drawing and rhythmic.' Nevertheless, they concluded that, 'Fundamentally our results lend support to the contention that there is some degree of unity in personality, that this unity is reflected in expression and that, for this reason, acts and habits of expression show a certain consistency among themselves.' There is a dearth of research on the use of body movement for identification and as a consequence we have mentioned studies which may have a bearing either directly or tangentially upon this issue.

Most of the descriptions encountered in police work do mention non-facial aspects of the individual. Details of age, height, weight and clothing are often disseminated, though at present movement details are rarely given except in extreme cases (e.g. 'suspect walks with a limp') – perhaps because, as Tagiuri and Petrullo (1958) note, 'We seldom describe the sheer sequence of the bodily movements of a person.' However, we do possess quite a large vocabulary for describing the more static aspects of a person such as those just listed. Unfortunately few studies have ever been published concerning the discriminatory powers of even these commonly mentioned characteristics.

AGE

Intuitively it seems that observers are reasonably accurate when judging the age of others and Kogan, Stevens and Shelton (1961) found that even four-year-old children could correctly rank photographs of people as a function of judged age. However, in their analysis of the testimony of 20,000 real-life witnesses Frank and Frank (1957) found the average inaccuracy of the age judgments to be eight years, and the case of 'The Cambridge Rapist' suggests that witnesses can sometimes judge ages inaccurately, especially if the face is concealed.

HEIGHT

Wilson (1968) noted that five groups of his students could accurately judge his height (to within one inch) when he was no longer in view. However, having introduced an accomplice to the groups (once as a undergraduate, to the second group as a research student, to the third as a lecturer, to the fourth as a senior lecturer, and to the fifth as a professor), it was found that their judgments of the accomplice's height once he had left the room, were significantly related to his ascribed status. The group means for estimated height, as a function of increasing status were 5 feet $9\frac{1}{2}$ inches, 5 feet 10 inches, 5 feet 11 inches, 5 feet $11\frac{1}{2}$ inches, 6 feet $\frac{1}{2}$ inch ($p < 0.001$), and the accomplice's actual height was 6 feet 1 inch. Dannenmaier and Thumin (1964) observed a similar effect though their experimental design was rather poor. These results can be seen as an example of the operation of stereotypes, a factor which was discussed in Chapter 3. However, neither Rump and Delin (1973) nor Lerner and Moore (1974) found an effect of ascribed status upon judged height though the latter authors did notice that their observers underestimated the perceived man's height by a mean of 2 inches (he was 5 feet 10 inches). As a basis for such stereotypes Wilson and Nias (1976) draw attention to a survey of Pittsburg University graduates' careers which was conducted by the *Wall Street Journal*. Here it was found that tall men (i.e. over 6 feet 2 inches) received significantly higher salaries than men less than 6 feet tall. They also note that every President of the USA elected since the turn of the century has been the taller of the two candidates (Jimmy Carter being an exception). It is noteworthy that in Wilson's (1968) study all the estimates of the accomplice's height were underestimates (in reality he was quite tall). It is possible that when an observer is asked to recall certain details which are not readily available in his memory he may employ schema-generated perceptions or known population norms. This might not be a bad thing, however, because if details of an attribute (e.g. height) cannot be recalled then it is likely that they were not abnormal in the first place and thus resorting to the stating of norms could in fact result in accuracy.

Dillon (1962) noted that individuals tended to overestimate their own heights. (It is not known whether this is merely an egocentric reaction in our culture where being tall can be thought of as desirable.) If all observers err in the same manner when making such judgments then perhaps this consistency will not necessarily result in poor recognition if the utilization of the data is prone to the same error. But if idiosyncratic stereotypic reactions are employed (as mentioned in Chapter 3) things may not be so consistent. Dunaway (1973) investigated in a non-stress situation the effects of the height and sex of the observers upon their height estimation of others. The observers are reported to have in general underestimated the height of tall people and overestimated the height of short people with the former being more prone to error than the latter. Of greater interest is the finding that shorter observers underestimated heights more so than did taller observers, and vice versa, with the cross-over point from under- to over-estimation being at approximately the average female height (65 inches) for female observers and at the average male height (68 inches) for male observers. Thus the general norms for the population may have been influencing the observers' height estimates together with the effects of their own heights. The first author has observed the former of these effects in several of his own studies (reports of which are in preparation), and the possibility of the latter effect is supported by the work of Williams (1975) who found a significant positive relationship to exist between observers' heights and their estimates of the height of an armed robber seen in a brief film. The taller the witness in Williams' study the taller was the criminal reported to be, and a similar relationship was noted for weight.

In a study conducted by Koulack and Tuthill (1972) it was noticed that when white students were shown various full-length photographs of a number of individuals their height estimates were influenced by the ethnic group to which they were informed that the individual belonged. (One wonders what the height estimates made by non-white observers would have been.) Many years ago Marks (1943) conducted an experiment along similar lines but here skin colour was the factor judged. Employing a seven-point rating scale it was found that light-skinned negro students rated medium-dark individuals as 'darker than average', whereas dark-skinned negro students rated the same individuals as 'lighter than average'. This significant effect could be the result of many factors, one of which might be the self-referential act of being normal, i.e. the observers believed themselves to be normal or average and so anyone lighter (or darker) than they must be above or below average. Bailey, Shinedling and Payne (1970) suggests that obese individuals believe the average person to be fatter than do thin people.

These findings suggest that aspects of the observer are important in person description. Are most people 'tall' to the man who is 5 feet 2 inches? It is also possible that other aspects of observers can influence what is recalled. A hairdresser may notice and therefore recall details of hairstyle whereas a clothes designer may remember only things about the clothes an individual wore. There may be racial differences here. Perhaps the police should note down a description of the witness as well as the witness's description of the suspect.

CLOTHING

Clothing often forms a large part of any person's description though, as Allen (1950) points out, any thinking criminal will make an attempt at disguise. There are many circumstances when this is not possible and though a wanted person may soon discard the clothes worn at the time of the relevant incident, it is likely that he will adopt attire of a similar style. A person's choice of apparel is rarely arbitrary (Argyle, 1969) and several studies support the contention than an individual will consistently adopt similar types of clothing whilst the actual garments worn may vary slightly (Aiken, 1963; Bull, 1975; Compton, 1962). With this in mind the dissemination of details of clothing may prove useful, as it does when it reminds someone of specific attire. Simmonds, Poulton and Tickner (1975) provided observers with photographs of the 'wanted' person who would appear in a film of a street scene. For some observers the wanted person was wearing the same clothes in both the photographs and in the film but for other observers the clothing in the photographs was different from that in the film. Not surprisingly those observers who saw the same clothing in both film and photographs made significantly more correct identifications than those who did not.

This chapter demonstrates that little information is at present available concerning person identification by visual, non-facial cues. However, this very paucity of data provides much scope for future investigations. Several topics have been mentioned and these together with studies of gestures and postures may be worth following up. Hewes (1957) noted that there are cross-cultural differences in posture, and Knapp (1972) in body movement. There are probably consistent sub-cultural differences as well. Fast (1971) believes that greater knowledge about body language will improve our recognition skills and he notes that, 'By specific gestures a talented mimic can tell us not only what part of the world the portrayed individual comes from but also what he does for a living,'

One of the major problems facing research in this area is our lack of an appropriate vocabulary with which to describe body movement. Some attempts have been made to improve the situation (Birdwhistell, 1971; Kendon, 1971; Garrett and Kennedy, 1971) but much still needs to be done. Some verbal communication of the details of visually perceived movement is possible (Carmichael, Roberts and Wessell, 1937) but it might be more worth while to develop graphical, photographical or mechanical techniques.

VOICE

The study of voice recognition also suffers from a lack of an appropriate descriptive vocabulary. Most identification situations involve the observer using visual cues but there are some instances when both visual and verbal information is available, and others when only verbal clues exist. In obscene telephone calls, for example, often the only possible method of identifying the speaker is by his voice. Similarly in kidnap cases information concerning the kidnapper's voice is sometimes made available by him over the telephone. In such situations when a suspect is in the hands of the police a voice-matching exercise may be entered into. Here a witness may be asked whether the suspect's voice is the same, or resembles, the criminal's, or a machine may be employed in an attempt to answer these questions if a record (e.g. a tape) of the original criminal voice is available.

The Devlin Committee, which reported to the Home Secretary in 1976 its findings in respect of the evidence of identification in criminal cases, stated that in connection with person recognition by voice, 'as far as we can ascertain there has been no scientific research into this question'. We have already commented on this report elsewhere (Bull and Clifford, 1976) and it is true to say that this committee did not avail itself of much of the psychological information which is available on the topic of person identification. There has in fact been quite a lot of research conducted on voice recognition especially in connection with the spectrographic analysis of speech and this topic will be examined once other studies of voice recognition have been described.

As early as 1937 psychologists began their examination of the reliability of voice identification. McGehee (1937) was concerned with attempting to answer the questions: (i) 'what is the influence of time-interval upon memory for voices?'; (ii) 'what is the effect of increasing the number of voices heard in a series in which occurs a voice to be subsequently recognized?'; (iii) 'to what extent is a voice recognized as having been heard previously when disguised by a change in pitch?'; (iv) 'are there sex differences in the recognition of voices?' The experimental procedure involved groups of students listening to an adult reading aloud a paragraph of fifty-six words from behind a screen. Each of the readers was unacquainted with any of the listeners and none had a noticeable dialect or speech defect. In all there were 31 male and 18 female readers, there being a total of 740 listeners. All the groups of listeners were tested for voice recognition after time intervals ranging from one day to five months. In the recognition situation each of five readers successively read aloud the initial passage and the listeners were required to note down which of the five readers they had heard previously. For listeners who initially heard only one reader McGehee observed 83, 83, 81 and 81 per cent accuracy for time intervals of one, two, three and seven days respectively. After an interval of two weeks performance dropped to 69 per cent and after a further week to 51 per cent. Intervals of three and five months led to accuracy scores of 35 and 13 per cent respectively. Thus, it was concluded that with the passage of time, 'there is a general trend towards a decrease in percentage of listeners who were able to correctly recognize a voice the second time it is heard.'

During the initial part of the experiment some listeners heard not one voice but several and it was found that the more voices heard initially the more difficult was it to recognize subsequently any one of them (83 per cent accuracy for the case in which only one voice was heard initially, down to 50 per cent when more than three voices were heard initially). As noted above, the case in which only one voice was heard initially resulted in 83 per cent recognition on the next day when on both occasions the voice demonstrated its normal pitch. If, however, on the second day the voice was disguised by a change in pitch then only 67 per cent of the listeners recognized it.

Concerning sex differences, McGehee found men to be better voice recognizers than women (84 per cent accuracy vs. 59 per cent), but that male voices were no better recognized than were female voices (72 per cent vs. 71 per cent). Significant interactions were noted in that men were very good at recognizing female voices (96 per cent) but were not so good with male voices (73 per cent), whereas women were better with male voices (72 per cent) than with female voices (47 per cent).

In 1973 Bartholomeus examined voice identification by nursery school children five months after the start of the school year. She played to two groups of children, aged four and five years, tape-recorded speech samples obtained from the classmates and teachers. Each child was provided with a series of recorded voices and was required to identify each speaker in turn having been told that they were classmates or teachers. In one condition the stimulus consisted of a two-sentence-long speech sample and the child was required to say out loud the name of the person who had provided the speech sample. In another condition the same stimuli were given but the identification response required the child to pick out from an array the photograph of the speaker. The third condition provided speech samples that were played backwards and each child was asked to name the speaker. In a fourth condition each child was required to name the classmates and teachers in the photographs shown to him. Four teachers also acted as subjects in this study. For each child (and teacher) the face-naming task produced the highest accuracy score (97 per cent for the children and 100 per cent for the teachers). In the voice-to-face-matching task the children's accuracy score dropped substantially to 58 per cent and that of the teachers to 81 per cent. Bartholomeus pointed out that errors in this task cannot be attributed to failures at picking out the right face having correctly identified the voice because the children were almost perfect at face naming. Scores in the voice-naming task were similar (56 per cent for the children and 68 per cent for the teachers) and again Bartholomeus argues that here the errors made cannot be attributed to the unavailability of appropriate verbal labels (i.e. not knowing the names of the children in the class). As one might expect the speech played backwards occasioned the lowest identification scores (41 per cent for the children and 63 per cent for the adults) but such a level of accuracy is still greater than could be expected by chance alone and this led Bartholomeus to claim that, 'These results demonstrate substantial ability in the identification of voices from samples of unintelligible speech.'

At first glance it might seem surprising that the teachers were not perfect at identifying the voices of children with whom they had interacted for several hours a day for five months. However, it is important to note that the children were all of a similar age and therefore their voices would be quite similar to one another, at least in pitch. Bartholomeus noted that one or two voices were consistently easily identified in any condition and some others were constantly mis-identified. She believes that the inaccuracies in the voice-naming and voice-to-face-matching tasks can be attributed to inefficient processing of available auditory cues, and that this may be because the auditory cues concerning an individual's identity are normally analysed during or after the processing of simultaneously presented linguistic information whereas purely non-verbal visual cues are processed immediately. That is, when a voice is heard the input is analysed for the meaning of the words being spoken and the act of doing this may to some extent prevent details of the actual voice being remembered. (A similar point was made in Chapter 4.)

Bartholomeus noted that some listeners were reliably much better at speaker identification than were others with the teachers tending to be most accurate of all. However, since the best teacher's score was equalled or exceeded by some of the children on each test, it can be concluded that at least some of these 4- and 5-year-olds were as accurate as were adults at voice identification. This being the case Bartholomeus believes that, 'a lack of substantial improvement in speaker recognition after early childhood would be consistent with the adoption of a perceptual strategy which optimizes efficient decoding of linguistic information by relying on vision, rather than audition, for information concerning an individual's identity.' The results in this experiment also provided evidence of correct recognition of the sex of the speaker in cases of incorrect identifications. Bartholomeus takes these findings to indicate that speaker identification involves a hierarchical sequence of judgments in which absolute identification is preceded by categorization of voices with respect to different variables such as age or sex. How this may be done was not commented on and Bartholomeus believes that, 'the cues used by listeners when identifying voices remain largely unknown.' Within the confines of this experiment there was no doubt that voice identification was more difficult than face identification. However, to what extent this difference was a function of the testing situation is not known.

There have been some attempts to examine the utility of possible identification cues in speech. Scherer (1974) tried not so much to determine which cues are used in identification but to see whether listeners could agree in their attribution of certain voice quality characteristics to various voices. In his study a large number of voice attributes was employed rather than the more restricted number relating to energy and frequency which are employed in electroacoustic equipment measures. In his experiment Scherer played to listeners twenty-second speech samples of various adult male speakers. Each sample was from only one speaker but it consisted of a number of randomly arranged mini-samples, each of less than one second duration so that the resultant sample conveyed minimal meaning in terms of containing intelligible words. Each listener was required to rate each voice for such things as pitch, height and range, loudness, breathiness, creak, glottal tension and nasality, on a thirty-five-item voice quality attribute rating form. The listeners consisted of the speaker himself, three of his acquaintances, six experienced phoneticians who were deemed to be expert judges, and groups of adult females who were considered to be lay judges. Each listener was provided with two minutes worth of voice sample per speaker by continuous repetition of each twenty-second speech sample. Inter-agreement was fairly high for the ratings by the expert judges, especially for judgments of loudness, pitch height and pitch range, and several of the attributes being judged were found to be interrelated. However, when the ratings from the expert judges were compared with measures of the speech samples obtained by the use of a computerized filter-bank spectrum-analyser (i.e. average energy, energy variation, average pitch and pitch variation) very few significant correlations were found. The ratings by the expert judges were also compared with those of the lay judges and some measure of agreement was found, especially for pitch and loudness. This led Scherer to view pitch and loudness as the most powerful vocal dimensions affecting lay judgments. Neither the acquaintances nor the speakers themselves agreed with the expert and lay judges for ratings of the loudness, pitch or resonance of their friends' voices. Scherer points out that, 'The lack of strong correspondence between self and acquaintance ratings of voice quality and expert ratings raises the interesting question of the validity of self and acquaintance ratings of voice.' He believes that, 'It is possible that if one has been acquainted with a person for a long period of time and has heard that person's voice in many situations, the resulting wealth of experience interferes with the accuracy of the description of the voice.'

It may be worth while to bear Scherer's comments in mind when assessing the findings of studies such as that of Bartholomeus (1973). However, the voice stimuli provided in Scherer's study could seem so artificial as to make the study of little value to those interested in the identification of persons by the way they speak. Nevertheless, Scherer did find that there was a difference in voice quality between German and American speakers and this may have some bearing upon the possibility of regional dialects playing a role in person identification. There seems little doubt that the voices of various people do differ reliably from each other since we often appear able, for example, to recognize the voice of someone on the telephone even when they do not announce who they are. People from different walks of life and different parts of the country do speak in a variety of ways and it can be shown that stereotype judgments are made on the basis of speech (Mulac, Hanley and Prigge, 1974).

Bortz (1970) investigated how one's own voice may influence the judgments of the voices of others and his experiment is an interesting parallel to those of Marks (1943) concerning skin colour judgments and Dunaway (1973) on height judgments mentioned previously. Audiotapes were made of students each reading three texts. Each reader judged his own voice and the voices of others on a thirty-two-item rating scale. The voices were also rated on this scale by a number of psychologists. It was found that (i) raters with high-pitched voices judged others as having low-pitched voices, and vice versa; (ii) raters with strongly dynamic voices overestimated existing differences of expression in the voices of others; whereas (iii) raters with less dynamic voices underestimated such differences. The rater-ratee interaction was concluded to be such that the closer a rater identifies with the voice of the ratee, the less suitable was his own voice as an objective standard of comparison.

Both Shipp and Hollein (1969) and Ptacek and Sanders (1966) showed that most people are able accurately to estimate the age of talkers from listening to their voices.

In an early and rather limited study Pollack, Pickett and Sumby (1954) played to seven listeners, for varying durations, the voices of men that they knew. It was found that the larger the speech sample the more accurate were the identifications, this effect being due to the greater speech repertoire evidenced in the longer samples since repetition of short samples did not increase the number of correct identifications. Whispered speech, which contains little pitch inflection, and which is of similar pitch for various speakers led to some correct identifications but far fewer than normal speech. Bricker and Pruzansky (1966) also examined the effect of stimulus duration and content upon talker identification. For the voices of people who worked together they found 98 per cent correct identifications when spoken sentences were provided, 84 per cent for syllables and 56 per cent for vowel excerpts. When the accuracy scores were plotted either against the number of different phonemes contained in the speech sample or against its duration the former was found to provide a better picture of the relationships than did the latter. Bricker and Pruzansky concluded that the improvement in identification with sample duration is due to an increased sample of the talker's repertoire being provided.

Murray and Cort (1971) also investigated the ability to identify speakers on the basis of the duration and repertoire of the speech sample. Twenty boys and girls aged 11 years from the same school class each provided speech samples which were to act as stimuli for the others. The samples consisted of a paragraph, a sentence or a sustained vowel. For the paragraph the children read aloud for twenty seconds, the sentence took five seconds to utter and the sustained vowel was obtained by asking each child to sustain the vowel 'a', as in the word 'farmer', for five seconds. One week after these recordings were made the children were divided into two groups, one group heard each of the recordings played once only and for each voice had to write down the name of the speaker, whereas for the other group each recording was played three times in succession before the next sample was played. A further seven days after these sessions the tests were repeated. No significant difference was observed between the correct identification scores of the listeners who had heard each sample only once and those who had heard each three times. Since the identification scores for the group which had heard each sample only once were very high for the sentence and paragraph speech samples (the mean for the sentence being 95 per cent and that for the paragraph being a few per cent higher), repetition of the samples for the other group of listeners could not be expected to boost the scores due to a 'ceiling' effect. However, this argument does not apply to the sustained vowel speech samples which led to only 48 per cent accuracy scores for the non-repetition group. Here there was room for improvement but two further repetitions of these samples did not improve the identification score of the group which received them. In the follow-up test the retest identification scores were very similar for each group in each condition except for the group which heard each speech sample once and here the vowel speech sample led to a drop in performance from 48 to 32 per cent accuracy. This follow-up test is not a test of delayed recall since during the two weeks of the experiment the children continued to interact in class. It merely serves as a replication of the first testing session, and it strengthens the conclusions of Murray and Cort that mere repetition of the same speech sample does not lead to any increase in identification accuracy scores whereas increasing the speech repertoire provided does so. They conclude that the repertoire available in a speech sample of a sentence in length is sufficient for identification performance to reach an asymptote and they conclude that for their subjects a fifteen-syllable sentence provided sufficient cues for voice identification. However, like the subjects in the study conducted by Bartholomeus, in this experiment the children had been together in the same class for at least several months. The conclusions which can be drawn from these experiments for the situations wherein recognition is required of a stranger who provided only one speech sample are tentative, but the adage of 'keep him talking' seems to have validity.

Kramer (1963) examined the judgments of personal characteristics and emotions based on speech. He provides a review of the studies which have investigated the existence of vocal stereotypes and it does seem that people reliably agree (sometimes with accuracy) upon such things as the personality, profession and physical appearance that they expect certain speakers to have. Thus, if such stereotypes exist they may introduce into the voice identification situation those factors referred to in Chapter 3. Kramer also cites a number of studies which suggest that an individual's emotional state can often be judged from his speech and it is important for any system of person identification based on voice that those aspects of speech which vary within an individual as a function of his mood be omitted from the recognition system.

VOICE IDENTIFICATION USING MACHINES

Though the police and judicial procedures for the recognition of persons by the way they speak are not as firmly laid down as they are for visual identification, the topic of identification by voice is one which has received quite a lot of attention from those wishing to develop electrical hardware to this end. Some success has been claimed for voice identification by spectrographic analysis and given the possibility that the number of meaningful ways in which voices may differ may be less than the number of ways in which faces differ then such advances are not surprising. Whereas at the moment mechanized person recognition using visual cues is still in its infancy, recognition by voice appears to have advanced a little further and may act as a guide for the development of visual systems and for their possible acceptance in legal settings.

Recognition by spectrographic voice analysis is based upon an electronic scanning of a speech sample which produces a visible amplitude/frequency/time display. This spectrogram can then be compared with other spectrograms to see if a match can be made. This matching is usually done not by the spectrographic machinery but by means of visual comparison of the spectrograms by a human, though mechanized systems of matching are being developed. The sound patterns represented on the spectrogram are the product of the energy displayed during speech and they are determined by the interplay between the individual's vocal mechanism (i.e. mouth cavity, soft palate, nasal and pharyngeal cavities, the vocal folds, etc.) and the coupling and placement of his articulators (i.e. the tongue, lips, jaw, etc.). As Cutler, Thigpen, Young and Mueller (1972) point out, the validity of this technique as a means of identification rests on the assumption that the sound patterns produced in speech are unique to the individual and that the spectrogram accurately and sufficiently displays this uniqueness. Further, as Wolff (1972) noted, a speaker recognition system should focus on those speech characteristics which cannot be modified or disguised by the speaker and which do not vary with health or mood.

Kersta (1962) was one of the first advocates of spectrographic voice analysis, claiming that voiceprint identification is closely analogous to fingerprint identification and that it is a more reliable method than handwriting comparisons. Fingerprint identification is widely accepted in the judicial setting but it is far less prone to the within-individual variations to which Wolff (1972) draws attention. In 1969 the Technical Committee on Speech Communication of the Acoustical Society of America asked some of its members to scientifically examine speaker identification by speech spectrograms (Bolt, Cooper, David, Denes, Pickett and Stevens, 1969). Their report concluded that the differences between identification by voice spectrograms and identification by fingerprints seemed to exceed the similarities and it was stated that, 'we doubt that the reliability of voice identification can ever match that of fingerprint identification'. Hall (1974) compares the reliability of fingerprints and voice-prints and concludes that, 'it is not valid to compare finger-prints with voiceprints.'

Kersta formulated the theory of invariant speech which holds that the spectral patterns of the same words spoken by two different people are more dissimilar than two such patterns resulting from the same person. He provided evidence that, at least to some extent, this theory is supportable. Trained spectro-gram examiners were able, with minimal error, to select from a small set of spectrograms those two which were most alike, knowing that a match existed somewhere in the set. Kersta's early experiments were criticized on the grounds that the number of spectrograms provided to the examiners for their search for a match was small and that the examiners were told that a match did exist. In a later experiment Kersta enlarged the samples and he also developed an automated system of voice identification (see Hennessy and Romig, 1971). This automated system counted the amplitude levels portrayed by the contour spectrogram at ten different locations on the spectrogram and a numerical code was devised for each voice sample. Fairly low error rates in identification were produced by this system if it was provided with speech samples five words in length or longer and these were due mainly to (i) the same word from the same speaker not always giving rise to the same code, and (ii) the same code resulting from two different people uttering the same word. For shorter speech samples the number of mismatches increased and this is in line with the studies cited earlier which suggested that a speech sample of about a sentence in length is the mini-mum required for attempts at identification. Recognition based on samples of isolated words is not so good and as Young and

Campbell (1967) have shown the lexical context of words is an important factor in spectrographic voice analysis. These researchers found that the identification error rate was far greater when the trained spectrogram examiners were provided with the spectrograms of the same words uttered in different sentences than when the same words were uttered individually and not in the context of a sentence.

One of the questions that has only infrequently been asked of spectrographic voice identification is whether it is any better than simple human identification by ear. It would seem rather a waste of time and money if this were not the case. Stevens, Williams, Carbonell and Woods (1968) found error rates of over 20 per cent for speaker identification employing spectrograms, but the persons who matched the spectrograms in this study were not extensively trained in the art as Kersta claims they should be. (It was noted that as the study proceeded the examiners' efficiency increased.) These examiners were required both to identify speakers by visually comparing spectrograms and also to identify speakers by simply listening to the tape recordings on which the spectrograms were made. It was found that the identification performance accuracy from aural comparisons was far higher than that resulting from the visual comparison of spectrograms (94 vs. 79 per cent at the end of the study), and that the time taken to arrive at the identifications was less for the aural input. Overall not only did the aural tests lead to better performance at the beginning of the study they also were the ones which derived the greatest improvement with practice. Further, for the aural information the length of utterance required for identification was shorter than that required by the spectrographic comparisons. Individual differences in accuracy between the identifiers were noted as was their confidence in their identifications. Stevens *et al.* concluded that 'differences between spectrograms of different talkers were much less apparent than the heard differences in the aural tests', and that, 'Authentication of voices is much poorer on a visual basis than on an aural basis'. This suggests that spectrographic voice analysis may certainly be no better than comparing the same voices by ear. (Stevens *et al.* also found 'at least weak evidence that a voice that is distinctive to listen to also has a distinctive spectrographic pattern.') Hecker (1971) stated that, 'whether future visual tests will provide lower error scores than future aural tests is debatable. ... The question about the perceptual bases of speaker recognition and their acoustical correlates remains largely unsolved.'

Many people have been sceptical about the claims made by the proponents of the accuracy of spectrographic voice identification and until a few years ago evidence based on such procedures was ascribed little status. However, as Cutler *et al.* (1972) reported, a study by Tosi does lend some support to Kersta's view. Not only were Tosi's results similar to those of Kersta for the matching-in-sample test, but also tested were the accuracy and reliability of experiments employing a more realistic identification format. Cutler *et al.* point out that the original matching-in-sample tests are not true 'identification' tests but involve simple 'similarity' judgments. In such tests all the examiner is required to do is find the sample in the set which best matches the spectrograph in hand, whereas in identification the examiner(s) has to be sure that two spectrographs are not only somewhat similar but are similar enough to have definitely come from the same speaker even when he has no prior knowledge of whether or not a true match exists in the sample provided.

Tosi, Oyer, Lashbrook, Pedrey and Nash (1972) employed both matching-in-sample and realistic identification tests and the speech samples contained less than ten words. A number of samples were obtained from each speaker and for some speakers a considerable time elapsed between the providing of the speech samples. Further, not all samples included the vocalization of identical sentences though the sentences did have some words in common. Realism was added to the study by recording the voices in three different ways. These were either directly into a tape recorder in a quiet setting, or via a telephone in a quiet or noisy situation to the tape recorder. A speaker population of 250 students was employed and these were selected to have no speech defects nor strong regional dialects. Each of the twenty-nine examiners was given considerable training in the interpretation and matching of speech spectrograms.

Tosi *et al.* found that the matching-in-sample tests resulted in over 95 per cent accuracy and an average of 83 per cent accuracy was obtained for the trials wherein the examiner was not told whether a true match existed in the sample or not. The error rate of 17 per cent combines an 11 per cent false elimination rate (i.e. a match was in fact present but the examiner failed to make it) with a 6 per cent false identification (i.e. a match was present but the examiner made the wrong one, or a match was not in reality present but the examiner made one). Stevens *et al.* also found that matching-in-sample tests lead to much higher accuracy than 'open' tests.

Prior to the appearance of these results a number of courts in the USA had held spectrographic voice identification evidence as inadmissible because it was believed that the technique's reliability had not been sufficiently demonstrated. Subsequent to the appearance of Tosi's results the technique was deemed admissible by several courts but not without some discussion of the weaknesses of Tosi's study. Though Tosi *et al.* had employed a larger sample of speakers than had previous investigations, doubts were raised concerning whether his data contained as much inter-speaker and intra-speaker variability as any other possible group of speakers. It was believed that although the study appeared to be methodologically sound it just did not go far enough. Further, since the matching of the spectrograms was performed by eye it was viewed to be a purely subjective comparison which involved less scientific quantification than the polygraphic 'lie-detector' tests, the admissibility of which is still being debated (see Lykken, 1974) and there are a number of parallels between the judicial status of these two techniques.

Further problems for spectrographic voice analysis are the facts that no two examples of phonetically identical utterances from the same speaker are ever exactly alike and that different speakers can produce very similar spectrograms (Ladgefoged and Vanderslice, 1967). Thus any match between two voice spectrograms can never be exact but can only involve a probability of having come from the same speaker and thus error is introduced. This question of probability is one which has always been a problem in legal settings. However, we hope that given the information provided in this book it is now realized that *all* evidence contains a degree of probability. A person's face seen twice *never* provides the same visual input to the observer. No two fingerprints are ever the same. Even your house has changed shape since you last saw it. Over and above these changes in the stimuli being perceived are the changes in physical viewing position of the observer, his mood and expectancies. The important question is whether the error inherent in any recognition technique is acceptable or not. A further criticism of Tosi's study was that none of his spectrograms came from subjects under psychological stress. Such stress may well be present in a criminal investigation and Cutler *et al.* suggest that it may have a significant effect upon speech production. Further, Hargreaves and Starkweather (1963) found that more identification errors were made when an individual's to-be-compared utterances were recorded on different days.

Edwards (1973) points out that the earliest judicial situations in which voiceprint evidence was admitted were those involving (i) the determination of probable cause, a point in criminal proceedings where 'incompetent' evidence can traditionally be used (e.g. the issuing of an arrest warrant) or (ii) the use of voiceprint information in a secondary role in the process of proof. Greene (1975) draws attention to the fact that in Tosi's study the greatest type of error involved the spectrogram examiners failing to make a match when in fact one existed. He takes this to mean that the use of spectrograms will more often result in the guilty going free than in an innocent person being accused, and he points out that, 'this technique has resulted in the elimination of far more criminal suspects than have been positively identified.' He concludes that,

> Criticisms of the Tosi study are grounded largely upon misunderstandings about the sophistication and knowledge-ability with which juries arrive at verdicts, the difference between the admissibility of evidence and the weight to be given evidence by factfinders in our legal system, the similarities and differences between voiceprint identification and other forensic disciplines such as fingerprint and handwriting identification, and the proper application of legal standards to the admissibility of scientific evidence. Thus it is not surprising that the overwhelming number of jurists at both the trial and apellate level who have considered the issue have concluded that voiceprint identification has reached the standard of scientific acceptance and reliability necessary for its admissibility into evidence.

Block (1975) provides interesting anecdotal accounts of many legal trials in which the admissibility of voiceprint evidence played a part and in which scientists from various backgrounds argued either for or against its validity. Whether such evidence was finally admitted was a function of many factors including the nature of any other evidence, the type of crime, the expert witnesses and the US state in which the court was located. At the present time such evidence is still not widely accepted and the current status was well summed up by one Judge McGuire who concluded that, 'the voiceprint process requires substantial additional research before it is accepted by the scientific community, let alone admissible by the legal community' (Block, p. 67).

To sum up, spectrographic voice analysis, just like any other sort of evidence, can never conclusively prove guilt. However, it can sometimes be used to establish a high likelihood of guilt. Such an act requires not merely that two spectrograms (the perpetrator's and the suspect's) be deemed to have come from the same person when only these (or a few others more) are compared by an expert. What needs to be established is that one, or preferably more, experts can reliably pick out from a large number (say in excess of thirty) of spectrograms from different but similarly spoken people the one which best matches the sample provided by the perpetrator.

At present it seems that not all courts agree on the admissibility of spectrographic voice identification evidence. Some deem it inadmissible whereas others view its shortcomings as insufficient to warrant ignoring it. Most seem to accept it in a way similar to their acceptance of visual identification evidence in that it is left to the court to note the possible weaknesses and unresolved questions that surround this technique. Both spectrographic voice analysis and polygraphic lie detection can be used not only by the prosecution but also by the defence as well. The use of these techniques to exclude persons from suspicion receives less criticism than does their use to positively identify an individual. It is rather rare for criminal guilt to be assigned solely on the basis of such techniques and at the moment they are employed mostly during the investigative stage of enquiries, proof of guilt requiring other sorts of evidence.

Mechanized speech recognizers have had some success with a limited number of inputs from a small group of persons. If, for example, it was required that a door should open in the presence of a few specified persons then modern automated speech recognition systems are available which will respond to certain specified words spoken by these people if they have on previous occasions provided the machine with similar inputs for it to use in its matching task. It will respond to these people if they say the specified words in their usual manner. Martin (1974) presents evidence that in such situations 99 per cent accuracy of response can be achieved but he is quick to point out that this kind of situation is far removed from one wherein a machine can respond to (or match) any words spoken by any person. In 1974 he stated that, 'No universal systems have been developed up to now that can perform for most users with an accuracy sufficient to be useful.' Thus, though voice recognition can be achieved by some machines for a very restricted sample, if a large sample of different voices were presented then today's machines would almost certainly be confused by them. Consequently, given the present level of development of voice recognition (or matching) machines there is little evidence that they could be of much use in person identification, especially since recognition is a different task from identification. However, since a substantial amount of research is taking place on this topic there may be some major developments in the next ten years, and any such developments will need to realize that a human identifies speech not only by the acoustic information upon which today's machines rely but also by the grammatical and contextual cues that are available. Denes (1974) believes that, 'the [human] listener relies on contextual cues for satisfactory perception. Most automatic recognition devices of the past utilize acoustic cues only and they are therefore at a strong disadvantage compared to the human listener.'

The Devlin Report pointed out that questions of voice identification at present arise rarely but it acknowledged that this situation may change and therefore stated that, 'research should proceed as rapidly as possible into the practicability of voice identification parades with the use of tape recorders or any other appropriate method which, among other things, would have to take into account the dangers of disguising the voice and the extent of changes induced by stress.' We would not disagree with such a suggestion since stress can influence the voice (Hecker, Stevens, von Bismarck and Williams, 1968; Williams and Stevens, 1969).

One further problem facing the acceptance of identification by voice is the possibility that, as Bolt *et al.* (1969) noted, voices can be mimicked. Many professional entertainers are able to speak in a way which to our ears sounds very similar to the speech of the person they are impersonating and it should be remembered that it has not been shown that the human ear is any less sensitive than is a spectrograph. It is not unreasonable to suppose that an innocent individual could be wrongly convicted or 'framed' by his voice being mimicked. Hollein and McGlone (1976) report details of an experiment which examined the sensitivity of the voiceprint method to the effects of speakers purposely disguising their voices. Each of twenty-five speakers read aloud a passage first in their normal voice and then they were instructed to do the same again this time 'disguising their voices in any way they chose except by whispering or using a foreign dialect'. Thus two speech samples similar in lexical content were provided by each speaker. The spectrogram examiners were 'familiar with the voiceprint method of speaker identification'. Each examiner was required to match in turn each of the twenty-five disguise exemplars with one of the 'normal voice' spectrograms. It was observed that, 'even skilled auditors such as these were unable to match correctly the disguised speech to the reference samples as much as 25 per cent of the time', and that,

> many of the subjects presented configurations for the disguise condition in which so many features were varied (relative to their normal production) that the two passages did not bear as much resemblance to each other as they did to productions by other subjects. Thus, except for the very small percentage of talkers who were relatively unsuccessful in disguising their voices (even they were misidentified nearly one-half of the time), these groups were able to disguise their voices, in such manners, that their identification by the voiceprint technique became little more than a matter of chance.

Hecker (1971) concluded his literature survey by pointing out that,

> In speculating on possible reasons for the superiority of listeners over machines in recognizing speakers, it is well to

remember that even the most naive listener has lived in a speech environment for a considerably longer period of time than any machine. The experience he has thus acquired cannot be readily defined and analogized.

6 Linguistic influences on memory for persons and events

Psychologists have accumulated evidence which suggests that language can 'bewitch' our memories for seen people and events, and that law enforcement agents must be careful not only that they ask the right questions but that they ask the right questions in the right way. This chapter will focus on the use of language by the 'witness', in the form of labels, and the use of language by those who are concerned to elicit an identification, a recall, or a description. As such this latter stress on 'elicitors' will be mainly in terms of language as questions: how they are phrased and how they are grouped and administered.

LANGUAGE AND MEMORY

The basic question is, does language in any way influence memory for visual material? This question, seen in its broadest perspective is part of what is called the Linguistic Relativity Hypothesis. This hypothesis suggests that language is a powerful determiner of perception and thought. The basic suggestion is that we dissect and interpret nature along lines laid down by our native languages. Slobin (1971) has suggested that there are currently two forms of this Whorf-Sapir linguistic relativity hypothesis: a strong form which states that aspects of language can determine thought, perception and memory, and a weak form that states that language can predispose people to think or act or perceive in one way rather than another. As Carroll (1964) points out, the linguistic relativity hypothesis has received little convincing support, and at best only the weak form carries any kind of conviction. In simulated real-life situations we will come to see that in fact language can influence what one thinks one has perceived and memorized about events and people, and that the choice of linguistic modes is a crucial consideration for police forces in the execution of their duty.

Before we discuss these real-life situations, however, let us try and clarify just if and how language and memory can interact. A number of studies have shown a correlation between verbal codability and visual memory, but correlation does not imply causality. Rather stronger, better evidence comes from experiments on the influence of labelling on memory for visual forms. For example Ellis (1968) and Santa and Ranken (1972) have shown that providing verbal labels aids recognition of nonsense (meaningless) shapes, when they are later presented for recognition, at least if the shapes are complicated and/or numerous. Most of the work on verbal labelling and recall or recognition of nonsense shapes has used only short delays between perceiving (learning) and recognition and as such there is a great deal of doubt over whether labelling can in fact aid long-term retention: Daniel and Ellis (1972) say that it can, but Santa and Ranken (1972) suggest it does not. While the controversy over nonsense material is not directly relevant, and thus will not be pursued further, what is of direct relevance is the possible explanations of the beneficial effect of labels in visual perception and memory. Ellis (1972) suggested verbal labels have their beneficial effect by focusing attention on distinctive stimulus features at the encoding stage while Santa and Baker (1975), on the other hand, suggest verbal labels aid retrieval. Thus if labels are beneficial they could be so as a result of two possible mechanisms. Ellis (1972) in his so-called Conceptual Coding Hypothesis would suggest that labels may have their effect by influencing the subject's encoding or scanning strategy, in such a way as to make him attend to specific features of the face at time of viewing. This view of labels has affinity to Gibson's (1969) pre-differentiation hypothesis of perceptual learning. The opposite view of the labelling effect comes from research based on Miller and Dollard's (1941) 'acquired distinctiveness of cues' hypothesis. This argument contends that labels make memory codes for different stimuli more distinct from each other by being part of the memory representation. In this case labels function mainly to aid retrieval by (i) increasing the distinctiveness of each stored trace, and (ii) providing more retrieval routes. This obviously has affinity with Paivio's (1971, 1976) dual coding hypothesis which argues that a concrete stimulus can be coded in both a visual and a verbal code and thus provide a greater number of retrieval routes at recollection.

While the theoretical locus of the labelling effect is both important and interesting a more immediate problem is whether in fact labelling goes on, and if it does, is it beneficial or harmful? We will look at these questions in terms of memory for meaningful material.

There is rather good evidence that verbal coding may play a significant part in remembering material more meaningful than nonsense shapes. A very famous study conducted in 1932 by Carmichael, Hogan and Walter shows this clearly. They presented a series of twelve ambiguous forms to two groups. To one of the groups, as they were being presented with these ambiguous forms, the experimenter presented a label, e.g. 'bottle' while to the other group the experimenter presented the label 'stirrup'. When subsequently required to reproduce the forms, subjects tended to distort their drawings in the direction of the appropriate label. This would seem to have direct relevance to the case where the witness is presented with a crime which, because of its speed, dynamism and inherent emotionality, can be likened quite easily to an 'ambiguous' situation or an ambiguous drawing. The label then attached to it, either by the perceiver himself, or by other witnesses, could very importantly distort the memory of the actual event. If this can be accepted then an important consideration arises, namely whether the distorting influence of a linguistic label comes at input or at output. A study by Prentice (1954) throws some light on this question. He showed that the effect of labelling was not present with recognition testing, suggesting that the labels did not affect storage of the visual trace but rather produced distortion at retrieval. Because recognition does not involve retrieval in the same way as does recall the distorting effect of labels was not seen in the Prentice study. Further support for the argument of labels having their effect at retrieval comes from Hanawalt and

Demarest (1939) who showed that labelling distortions can be produced when unlabelled figures are learned and subsequently cued by means of a label, e.g. 'Draw the figure that looked like a stirrup'. More recent research consolidates the effect verbal labels can have on visual memory. Cohen (1966, 1967) studied the effect of labels at recognition and found that when subjects were presented with an ambiguous figure (a circle with a 90° gap) and a label suggesting it was a clock with the hands at 'five to seven' or at 'ten to eight', both subsequent reproductions and recognitions (from a set of circles with gaps at different sizes) reflected the suggestion given during viewing of the initial circle. Thus subjects produce or 'recognize' larger gaps resulting from the label 'five to seven' being given. This reproduces the Carmichael *et al.* (1932) finding. The parallel here with the real-life study by Doob and Kirshenbaum (1973), outlined in Chapter 2 and to be discussed more fully below, is obvious. Cohen argued that in recognition as in reproduction, subjects use the labels to retrieve features from the representation of the stimulus in memory.

In the above studies 'reproduction' and 'recognition' have been used as if they are measuring the same type of memory. From our discussion in Chapter 2 it ought to be clear that they are not. *A priori*, it would seem that recall to a policeman taking down a statement or description, or a photo-fit constructor, because it uses verbalizations, ought to contain a greater possibility of a labelling effect than recognition which merely involves a perceptual matching. Cohen and Granstrom (1970) tested reproduction (recall) and recognition of irregular geometric visual forms after an interval of seven seconds, which was either filled with a visual distractor task (remembering sets of three faces) or with a verbal distraction task (remembering three names). The verbal distractor task interfered with the reproduction memory but not with the recognition memory, while the visual interference produced poorer recognition, but not poorer reproduction memory. Baddeley (1976) interpreted these results as showing that the recall of visual material depends on verbal coding whereas visual recognition is not dependent on verbal factors. However, this is at odds with the findings of Cohen (1966, 1967) and with the study by Doob and Kirshenbaum (1973). Real-life experiences and some experimental evidence do strongly suggest that verbal labelling occurs with visual experience and that these labels reappear at the time of trying to recognize the earlier seen object. While we will be discussing the possible effects of labelling on face recognition (both real-life faces and schematic faces) it may be worthwhile here citing the conclusion drawn by McKelvie (1976) in a study of recognition of faces which were either easy or hard to label: 'The major conclusion emerging [from this experiment] is that verbal labels appear to serve a dual role in recognition memory ... they guide the subjects examination and encoding of the stimulus during viewing and serve as mediators in the memory representation.'

In the light of what has been discussed above a safe summary may be the one proposed by Santa and Baker (1976) that, 'language in the form of labelling exerts a strong influence on the organization and retrieval of nonverbal representations.' Now it may be the case that labels are only beneficial with abstract shapes, and when used with meaningful material they may become less useful (e.g. Davies, 1969; Kurtz and Hovland, 1953) or positively harmful (Bahrick and Boucher, 1968). This would have serious implications for face recognition if it were the case. Is it?

LABELLING AND FACE MEMORY

The work with multi-dimensional scaling shows that subjects can readily ascribe adjectives (labels) to seen faces. The important question is whether such labelling aids memory for faces? We looked briefly at this aspect of face research in Chapter 2 where we indicated that Frijda and Van de Geer (1961) believed that visual recognition of facial expression can be a function of verbal codability, but pointed out that little empirical evidence existed as to whether this was in fact the case. We also indicated that it was unclear where the effect was located – at input, storage or retrieval. Howells (1938) pointed out that subjects who were superior at naming details of facial photographs were not superior at recognizing them. Also Malpass, Lavigueur and Weldon (1973) found that training in giving verbal descriptions of faces did not improve visual recognition performance.

Two recent studies have addressed themselves to this question of whether recognition of a seen face is better if it can be labelled. McKelvie (1976) investigated the effects of labelling on the encoding and recognition of schematic faces. He presented easy-to-label and hard-to-label schematic faces which a previous study (McKelvie, 1973) had provided. From this previous study it would seem that the ease or difficulty of labelling a face is a function of brow and mouth configuration. (McKelvie (1973) indicated that rating of meaningfulness (how easy it was to find an adjective to describe the face) and the meaning (the adjective given to the face) were 'mainly a function of brow and mouth'.) He found that giving a label to a hard-to-label face produced better recognition than merely observing the hard-to-label face, and when sufficient care was taken experimentally, labels also aided recognition of easy-to-label faces. Thus labelling faces does seem to improve later recognition, at least with schematic faces. What about real-life faces presented in photographic form? Chance and Goldstein (1976) examined whether use of two kinds of self-generated verbal labels for faces was related to the accuracy of recognizing these faces one week later. One group of subjects were instructed, 'write some one thing about the face which you believe will help you recognize it when you see it again'. Another group of subjects were told to write, 'some one thing which the face reminds you of or looks like to you'. A third group were not given label instructions but were told to expect a one week delayed recognition test. A fourth group were simply asked to rate the pictured faces for age, but were not told of a delayed recognition test. In this experiment there was only a weak superiority for labelling over non-labelling, and only for the first group who used 'describe' labels. This result would be disappointing but for the fact that Chance and Goldstein (1976, note 2) indicate that a statistical test did in fact show a significant difference between Group 1 and Group 2 and that when another unreported, but highly similar, study was combined with this reported study the difference became even more marked.

Thus the evidence does suggest that labelling can improve later recognition of a seen face. While these two studies can be taken as evidence, albeit weak, for a beneficial effect of labelling on later face recognition a closer inspection of the McKelvie and Chance and Goldstein data provides more interesting, and possibly applicable, information. McKelvie (1976) showed that labels have their main effect by focusing attention on specific facial features during viewing, and that the labels may be stored along with the visual trace to be used at output. Also important is the fact that some of the results show that labels will only be effective if actively generated by the subject – a finding which we have argued to have important theoretical implications. The Chance and Goldstein study indicates that simply generating labels actively is not sufficient. The type of label actively generated is crucial (as shown by the difference between their Group 1 and Group 2). Usefully, Chance and Goldstein make some comment on the type of labelling that went on. They comment that they 'are struck by the undifferentiated nature of labels'. Responses like 'dark hair', 'looks studious', 'seems mean' seem unlikely to possess sufficient uniqueness to provide the subject with much advantage in later recognition of particular faces. This has important practical implications as we will see in the study by Doob and Kirshenbaum (1973). In both the above studies these investigators looked at faces and their labels and then at recognition of faces and recall of their labels. Neither study looked at the recall of the labels as an aid to recognition of faces. This is unfortunate because as we shall see below in crime episodes it may be a single, stereotypic, verbal response which is stored with a poorly perceived and therefore poorly registered face. At recognition the label may be used to recall a face, in order to match it to the line-up face. Doob and Kirshenbaum looked at this 'partial remembering' in a real-life case. Witnesses usually have to give descriptions of seen criminals before they are actually asked to recognize or identify him. Now following the work by Kay (1955) it would seem that if a witness says, 'Was rather attractive' then he will remember this description and feel committed to it. At recognition he will try to pick out the person who best fits this publicly given description. Thus what we have is a visual sighting, a verbal labelling and then a later visual recognition based on the remembered verbal label. The label can be the same but the two visualized people can be different. We will argue later that the composition of a line-up predisposes witnesses to this type of error. Doob and Kirshenbaum (1973) relate the case of Shatford who was accused of being one of two men who robbed a Canadian department store of $7,000. The cashier who was robbed immediately reported an inability to remember very much about the two people involved. Three things however emerged in her initial testimony: (1) the two robbers looked sufficiently alike to be brothers; (2) they were well dressed; (3) they were 'rather good-looking'. Three days later the witness helped compile a composite picture of the subjects. At this stage the cashier was reported to have said that she contributed nothing to the picture composition because she could not remember their facial features at all. However, she was able to pick out the accused from a line-up which consisted of the accused and eleven other people. How could the cashier pick out the accused while not being able to remember any of his physical characteristics? One possibility exists – a remembered label ('rather good-looking') could have directed 'recognition'. If the accused was the best-looking man in the line-up then he would be chosen (whether or not he was the actual thief). Doob and Kirshenbaum put this to the test by asking twenty females to rate the men in the police line up photo according to 'how good-looking you think each of them is'. The accused was rated the most good-looking! Twenty-one further students were then given the label 'rather good-looking' and asked, 'if this is all you could remember who would you choose?' Once again the suspect was chosen eleven times, and as a second choice a further four times. If chance alone was involved he would only have been selected twice!

The above sections of this chapter sought to make clear the relationship between language and memory under the heading of labels. We found that verbal labels helped memory for abstract shapes but found less effect with meaningful forms such as faces. Taken together, however, the few studies which looked at the effect of labelling faces on later recognition make it clear that further study should be undertaken. Evidence was educed to show that labels are used both to increase encoding of specific features and to aid retrieval. Most worryingly, it was suggested that because language can have an effect at both input and output, it could have rather important, traumatic effects in the sense of possibly perverting justice. We found this in a real-life court case, and an experimental analog of it.

Thus law enforcement agencies and witnesses themselves must be very conscious of and careful about how they employ labels.

The employment of appropriate labels can have beneficial effects at least in the laboratory in terms of improving memory as Bower and Karlin (1974) showed. They had subjects rate (implicitly label?) faces for either sex, honesty or likeability. The latter two types of rating produced much greater recognition accuracy when the faces were later re-presented for identification as previously seen. This is fairly similar to the type of processing engaged in by the cashier in the Shatford case, and may account for her recognition ability without the ability to describe specific details of the face. So once again it seems as if laboratory studies may give us understanding of the necessary conditions of eyewitness recognition, but they certainly do not provide understanding of the sufficient conditions. Simulation studies, approximating to real life, show that recognition accuracy drops drastically compared to laboratory performance levels; how much more must it drop in actual real-life incidents?

LINGUISTIC INFLUENCES AS QUESTIONS

If it can be accepted, with qualification, that subject-generated verbal input can affect, either positively or negatively, accuracy of recognition then it ought to follow that linguistic input from outsiders could also affect memory for seen events and people. This part of the chapter addresses itself to this possibility. The input from outsiders is usually in the form of questions. The interesting possibility then becomes do such questions influence our memories for the event we are being questioned about?

ANSWERS DEPEND UPON THE WORDING OF QUESTIONS

Psychologists, sociologists and philosophers are very much aware that the answer one gets back depends very much on the question one asks initially, but very few people are actually aware of just how subtle the influence of questions are, or how they operate in situations of person identification. The same question can take many different, and apparently trivial, forms. A very early study dealing with the influence of formal questions on memory for seen events is one by Muscio (1915) in which he presented a series of moving pictures to his subjects and then questioned them about some of the events they had just witnessed. He used eight forms of question of varying suggestiveness and tabulated the accuracy of the answers for each of these types. He found that the most reliable type of question was one which referred to the actual seeing of an event and which did not use either the definite article ('the') or a negative. Most importantly Muscio showed that the various forms of questions could be used to elicit desired answers from the witnesses. Hunter (1964) lists six main form of question. A determinative question is the least suggestive of all and is simply introduced by a pronoun or interrogative adverb: 'What colour was the car?' A completely disjunctive question forces the witness to choose between two specified alternatives: 'Was there a car at the scene?' This can only be answered by a yes or no. An incomplete disjunctive question offers a choice between two alternatives, but also allows a third possibility: 'Was the car black or white?' A fourth type of question is the 'expective' question which is suggestive because it is framed in a negative form: 'Was there not a car at the scene?' A stronger form of suggestion is the 'implicative' question in which the questioner implies the presence of something which was actually absent: 'what type of gun was it?' The last type of question that Hunter cites is the consecutive question or the follow-up question which is used to augment a suggestion which has been implanted by a previous question.

Over and above these six forms of question they can all be increased in potency for suggestion if the questions ask about whether certain things happened or were present rather than whether the witness saw or heard them. Within a specific question form a mere change of word can have a massive effect. Harris (1973) asked the simple question, 'How tall was the basketball player?' or, 'How short was the basketball player?' Subjects asked the former question gave an answer whose average was 79 inches, while the second group gave an answer whose average was 69 inches. In a replication experiment Harris asked subjects either, 'How long was the movie?' or, 'How short was the movie?' He got back average answers of 130 minutes and 100 minutes respectively. This shows rather clearly that the changing of one word in a question can have a large effect on the answer given, especially when the event or dimension being asked about is difficult to judge, e.g. height (see Chapter 2).

Another case where the wording of a question produced diverse estimates of a difficult-to-judge dimension was one by Loftus (1974). Loftus had 100 students view a short film sequence depicting a multi-car accident. Immediately after viewing the film the subjects were given a twenty-two-item questionnaire which contained six critical questions, three referring to items present in the film, and three referring to items not present. For half the subjects all the six critical questions began with the words, 'Did you see a . . . ?', for the remainder of the subjects all the questions began with, 'Did you see the . . . ?' *The* presupposes the presence of something, *a* does not. *The* questions produced a greater number of perceptions of non-present items than did the *a* questions.

In 1974 Loftus and Palmer presented a video film of a car crash and asked the viewers questions about it. The questions used were shown to influence the numerical estimate of speed of the colliding cars. The questions were identical in form except for the verb. All sentences comprised the following form: 'What speed were the cars going when they —— (into) each other?' The dash was filled by different verbs for different subjects. The verbs used were 'smashed', 'collided', 'bumped', 'hit' and 'contacted'. The numerical estimates of speed increased with the increased 'violence' of the verb.

These studies serve to show that the form and wording of an outsider's question can bias the way in which subjects access their stored visual memory. Can it also be shown that the type of question asked can actually alter the storage of memory traces? Loftus is again the chief experimentalist here. Her interest is in the influence of language on memory for fast moving, fairly complex events. The basic paradigm is to present a video film, then ask a series of questions and then, at a later date, ask another series of questions and compare answers to the second set of questions given by groups of subjects given different initial questions. The crucial manipulation is the first questionnaire which contains presuppositional type questions. The rationale is that if the subjects treat the first set of questions as new information then they will introduce this into their already stored memories, and so change this initial memory. At later recognition memory traces will thus be a composite of initial storage and effects due to intervening questions.

In the first experiment to be reported here a film was run for one minute in which a car was shown turning right while disregarding a stop sign, and causing a five car bumper-to-bumper pile up. A ten-item questionnaire was then administered. The first question asked about the speed of the car in one of two ways:

1 (a) 'How fast was the car going when it ran past the stop sign?'

or

1 (b) 'How fast was the car going when it turned right?'

The last question was identical for all subjects:

(10) 'Did you see a stop sign for the car?'

Subjects responded to question (10) by circling Yes or No. Fifty-three per cent of the group who received question 1 (a) said they had seen a stop sign, while 35 per cent of those subjects who had been given question 1 (b) answered 'yes', they had seen a stop sign. It is important to note in this experiment that the stop sign was actually present on film, and thus the differential rates of saying 'yes', they had seen a stop sign, for the two groups given different forms of question 1 admits of a number of explanations. Loftus (1975) argues that it could be the case that the persons who answered 'yes' had seen the stop sign and stored it, and question 1 (a) merely served to strengthen this storage. Alternatively, it could be argued that the person did not see the stop sign and thus had no stored memory of it, but when the question 1 (a) was asked the subject revisualized or constructed the scene as it must have been, and thus stored a stop sign as a trace. Thus when he answered question (10) he was reading off from a stored trace which was not the product of a visualization or perception, but was rather the outcome of a verbal input and the question which involved a stop sign. The way to sort out these two possible alternatives is to use presuppositional questions which refer to something *not* present in the film.

This was done by Loftus and Palmer (1974) in the study

referred to above which varied the verb used in the questions about speed of cars. These questions were used as 'priming' or 'distorting' questions, because one week later the subjects were brought back and, among other questions, were asked: 'Did you see any broken glass?' The number of sightings of broken glass increased with the vigour of the verbs used one week earlier. No broken glass appeared in the film! This strongly argues for the second alternative argument advanced above. The subjects could not have had an initial memory of broken glass because none appeared in the film. Thus a 'new' memory for a supposed visual event was laid down by a verbal question. This shows clearly the role of inferential processes in human memory because there is more chance of broken glass occurring as the severity of the car collisions increase. This research shows rather clearly the subtlety with which we are dealing in person and event identification: memory is no simple affair!

As further troubling proof of the possibility of falsification of eyewitness identifications by means of question, Loftus presented 150 students with a brief video film of an accident and then asked half the subjects to estimate the speed of the car 'as it passed the barn' and asked the other half to give a similar estimate but made no mention of a barn. There was no barn in the film. One week later all subjects were asked, 'Did you see a barn?' 17.3 per cent exposed to the initial barn question said 'yes', only 2.7 per cent of the group which had received the question which did not mention the barn said they had seen a barn.

It seems beyond doubt that the use of presuppositional questions can cause faulty memory. Presuppositional questions are all too easy to ask if one is dealing with a question of fact about which you have some theory – precisely the position Trankell (1972) argues characterizes the police interrogation of witness and suspect. Their use of presuppositional questions will be numerous but quite unintentional. But even if we could ensure that really conscientious consideration was exercised all would still not be well because it seems to be the case that if you ask a direct question and then repeat the question at a later date you still get memory distortion. Loftus (1975) quotes one study within which she asked one third of the subjects a presuppositional question, one third a straight question and the remaining third no question at all. The presuppositional group produced 29.2 per cent false memories; the straight questions 15.6 per cent false memories and no question produced 8 per cent false memories.

Most of the studies referred to above have looked at the · influencing of visual memory for seen events. Does the same hold true for perception of people? Loftus, Altman and Geballe (1975) showed fifty-six university students a three-minute portion of the film 'Diary of a Student Revolution' in which eight demonstrators disrupted a class in a relatively noisy but non-violent way, and then left. After seeing the videotape the students were given one of two questionnaires. The 'passive' questionnaire involved critical questions like, 'Did you notice the demonstrators gesturing at any of the students?' or 'Did the Professor say anything to the demonstrators?' The critical questions in the 'active' questionnaire contained questions like, 'Did you notice the militants threatening any of the students?' or 'Did the Professor shout something at the activists?' One week later the subjects returned and answered another questionnaire. The critical questions tested whether the students given the active or the passive initial questionnaire would rate the incident as noisy or quiet, peaceful or violent, whether the demonstrators were pacifist or belligerent, and whether the students were sympathetic or antagonistic. The group who had received the initial active questionnaire rated the demonstration as more noisy/violent, more belligerent and more antagonistic than did the students who initially received the passive questionnaire. More relevant still is another experiment by Loftus (1975) in which she showed that the memory for the number of criminals in an incident could be influenced by the questions asked. They presented a three-minute videotape of a class disruption by eight demonstrators (see previous study). At the end of the film the subjects received one of two questionnaires which contained one critical question. Half the subjects received, 'Was the leader of the four demonstrators who entered the room a male?' The other half of the subjects received, 'Was the leader of the twelve demonstrators who entered the room a male?' One week later a questionnaire was given with the question, 'How many demonstrators entered the room?' Witnesses who had been given the 'twelve demonstrators' question one week earlier responded, on average, with 8.85; those witnesses given the 'four demonstrators' question initially answered, on average, 6.40.

These studies thus show that memory for atmosphere and the number of criminals can be altered by questions. What about actual actions or appearance? It could be argued that questions should be less harmful with people and their actions. It seems that they are not. Once again research casts grave doubts on the independence and autonomy of visual and verbal memory. We have already discussed 'unconscious transference' (Chapter 2) in the case of the ticket collector who falsely accused a sailor of being a criminal because of a similarity of situations, i.e. a train station (Houts, cited in Wall, 1965). There are frequent cases in law where witnesses have confused which person was doing what when, or whether person A was at point B at time C, or at some other time altogether. We will now look at studies which show this quite clearly and the power of language or questions to exacerbate it. Miller and Loftus (1976) presented twenty-six students with 20 photographic slides for 3 seconds each. Each slide depicted one of five persons, engaged in one of four different activities such as blowing up a balloon, reading a book, solving a jigsaw puzzle. Thus each model was seen four times doing four different activities. No two models were ever seen doing the same activity. The slides were then followed by ten minutes of filler activity which was designed to (a) cause delay between viewing and trying to remember the people and their activities, and (b) to prevent subjects rehearsing the content of the slides. Following this filler activity a slide was shown of one of the five persons (now doing nothing) and a question was asked such as, 'What colour of balloon was he blowing up?' In certain cases person and questioned activity were appropriate, in the sense that the slide person had actually been doing the activity questioned. On other occasions the activity questioned was inappropriate to the slide person – he had not been seen doing that activity. The third phase of the experiment involved showing twenty slides and asking subjects to say if they had been presented before. Six were old, six were new (not seen before), eight were of models doing something different from what they had been seen doing before. Questions asked in phase 2 suggested to the subjects that four of the eight slides, where the model was doing something never seen before, were old or had been seen before, whereas no false suggestion had been made about the remaining four unseen slides. True recognition of seen slides was 88 per cent. False recognition of 'suggestion slides' was 69 per cent. False recognition of non-suggestion slides was 48 per cent. False recognition of new slides was only 3 per cent. Thus by asking a witness a leading question and indicating a specific person it is possible to induce a witness to testify later that he had seen that person doing something which was actually not true.

Now it can be argued that this experiment as it stands is a little complex or difficult. Five people each doing four things produces a fairly complex permutation, and therefore a difficult memory task, but it is not too discrepant from crime episodes which involve gangs. However, to avoid this possible accusation Miller and Loftus performed a second, less complex, experiment. Subjects saw six models each doing one thing only. All the 100 subjects heard a tape recording of a story concerning these six college students. As each of the six characters was mentioned a slide of him was shown for approximately two seconds. All the subjects heard the following story:

> Of Jim Fisher, the valedictorian of his class, it is commonly said that he gives a misleading initial impression. Many of his classmates find him, on first acquaintance, to be a quiet, somewhat distant person who is more measuring than gregarious. 'It is often said of Jim that he is aloof and calculating', says Howard Leland, who is a long term friend of Fisher's. Some people resent this. In fact one day last week several of the guys on the debate team including Robert Dirks initiated an argument with Fisher for seemingly no reason at all. They were all probably in a rotten mood and wanted someone to pick on. Steve Kent was the worst of the bunch; he went too far this time. When Fisher started yelling back, Kent picked up a heavy paper weight and threw it at Fisher, hitting him on the side of the head. Fisher fell over. Two people had witnessed the whole event. Sam Tappin ran to the nearest telephone to call an ambulance. He had trouble speaking coherently because he was so nervous about what had happened. David McCoy rushed over to help Fisher. The rest of the guys had already run away.

The slides of the people mentioned on the tape were each depicted in one visual situation. Fisher was shown walking past the auditorium. Howard Leland was shown driving by the auditorium. Robert Dirks was shown walking up to the auditorium, wearing a small brown hat. Steve Kent was shown with a paper weight in his hand, and so on.

After hearing the tape and viewing the slides all subjects participated in filler activities for forty minutes. The subjects were then asked ten questions about the original story one of which was critical. Half the subjects were asked, 'After the guy with the hat threw the paper weight at Fisher did he run away?' The other half of the subjects were asked, 'After the guy threw the paper weight at Fisher did he run away?' Note that the first question falsely implied that the person with the hat (Dirks) had thrown the paper weight. Three days later the subjects were shown six full face photographs – one of each of the six characters in the story and asked whether the person who had thrown the paper weight was amongst them, and which one was he. Of the fifty subjects who had been asked the question implying that the person with the hat committed the crime twelve chose the man with the hat. Of the fifty who had not been deliberately misled only three chose that person. This is a significant effect and indicates that a leading question can seriously distort memory for persons and their actions. Although Miller and Loftus do not stress the fact, it is worth pointing out that overall only 69 per cent picked out the correct man, and therefore 31 per cent picked out some-one else – and this only three days after near ideal listening and viewing conditions.

To summarize the studies so far. All the studies show that additional information (true or false) provided subsequently via questions can seriously distort and change memory for a previously seen event or person. Specifically, new information can alter the judgment about speed of vehicles, or severity of automobile accidents, can raise or lower the number of people said to be involved in a classroom distruption, and could increase the likelihood that non-existing objects would be recalled as having been seen. Suggestive questions can induce a witness to accuse a person of something someone else did, that is, to transfer the remembered action from one person to another.

So far then we have looked at language as labels and found it to be both a positive and a negative force. We then looked at language as questions and found it to be predominantly negative. A third important area is the overall style of questioning: whether it is better to allow people to freely construct their own accounts or for a list of questions to be produced which they have to fill in.

STRUCTURED VERSUS UNSTRUCTURED TESTIMONY ELICITATION

Alfred Binet, the famous French psychologist, was aware of the potential difference between these two modes of questioning as long ago as 1900. Basically Binet presented a picture and then at a later time asked for a description of it. This description was acquired in one of two ways: (i) report or narrative form; (ii) deposition or interrogative form. A report is elicited by merely asking the witness to tell, or write down, as much as he can recall, i.e. a free report. The deposition is based on a list of questions which, hopefully, covers all relevant aspects of the seen picture in Binet's case. Most early research on these two types of questioning procedure was European-based, stemming from Binet.

These two basic types of report structure can be assessed under at least three headings (Hunter, 1964): (1) range – the number of items measured; (2) accuracy – factual correctness; (3) assurance – degree of confidence by the witness that his recall is accurate and correct. Research has concluded that narrative reports are more accurate but less complete, while interrogative or depositions are more complete but less accurate. This has been reported by, among others, Gardner (1933), Marquis, Marshall and Oskamp (1972), Marston (1924), and Whipple (1909). No police officer or lawyer, however, uses these two forms of eliciting information in an either-or way, more frequently they are used consecutively, or in tandem. The question then arises, do the various methods of obtaining testimony differentially influence accuracy and completeness of recall? Several investigators have sought possible interactive effects typically employing both narrative and interrogative reports but changing the order for different groups of subjects. Thus when one group received narrative and then interrogative questioning while the other group received them in the opposite order, Cady (1924) found more accurate testimony when the narrative report was given first. Snee and Lush (1941) supported Cady's findings and also indicated that a narrative-interrogative order produced more correct responses, fewer 'don't knows', but no appreciable change in the frequency of incorrect responses. Whitely and McGeoch (1927) investigated the delay between completing one set of reports and then another, where delays were at least thirty days. They concluded that the narrative-interrogative order had a facilitative effect upon subsequent narrative recalls at delays of 30, 60, 90 and 120 day intervals.

Hunter (1964) maps out a number of the general conclusions that can be drawn. A completely accurate testimony is almost never achieved. One German investigator collected a total of 240 testimonies and found only five errorless reports and one error-less deposition. Even these errorless reports, however, are weak because while factually correct they lacked range, i.e. the witnesses were excessively cautious and only wrote down what they were absolutely certain of. There is no safety in numbers. Details which are incorrect may be reported by a majority of witnesses. Wall (1965) cites a number of cases where incorrect testimony has been offered by 13, 14, 17 and even 30 witnesses. These agreements in error occur specifically in such things as time estimation, sequence of events, and spatial location of people and objects. These tend to be schema-generated 'perceptual-memories' and conform to expectation and knowledge of norms, rather than to facts. Hunter quotes a study by Stern who showed the effect of expectation. During a lecture a man entered a room and asked if he could consult a book; the professor, aware of the contrived nature of the incident, said yes. The man read the book for some minutes while the class continued with the lecture. The man eventually left carrying the book. A week later the students were asked to retell, via a questionnaire, what they could remember about the events and the man. There were many errors of omission and commission but of chief interest was the response to the question, 'What did the man do with the book?' The majority wrongly said that he had replaced it on the shelf. A strictly enforced rule of the classroom was that no book should ever be removed. Thus a schema based upon incorporated rules about books had caused a vast majority of students to declare unhesitatingly, and in all sincerity, that they had seen the man return the book to the shelf.

Generally speaking an interrogative report produces greater range but less accuracy. The proportion of inaccurate items is something like a tenth for narrative reports and a quarter for interrogative. Why should this be so? In free report the subjects will report only what he remembers and is sure of, while under interrogative report he will be asked questions to which he has no relevant memory, but because he is being asked by an authority figure an answer is likely to be given; also, by the very fact of being asked a question the implication is that he ought to know the answer, and is considered capable of giving it. When an answer has been given, however uncertainly and haltingly, it becomes a 'fact' and the witness leaves all doubts behind and accepts his output as the outcome of genuine recall, and this is especially the case if the interrogator seems pleased with the answer and goes on to ask further, consecutive, or follow-up, questions. While we will discuss children as eyewitnesses in Chapter 7 it is worth pointing out here that children are inferior to adults in both the range and accuracy of their testimony, i.e. they give fewer items and what they do give is more likely to be inaccurate. In part, as Hunter points out, this is due to their poorer ability to observe, to understand and to use language, but in part it is due to their greater suggestibility, at least in terms of accuracy. They are particularly likely to answer leading questions in accordance with the suggestion they carry. Thus Stern (1924) has estimated that 7-year-old children are misled by some 50 per cent of leading questions, with 18-year-olds misled by only 20 per cent of such questions.

The correlation or positive relationship between recognition accuracy and confidence of reliability is very low or non-existent. Less error is found in sworn testimony than in unsworn testimony but inaccuracies still remain in the former, especially as the time between viewing and recognition tests increases. Stern (1910, 1939), Whipple (1909) and Weld (1954), while indicating generally that testimony is rarely accurate, suggest that when subjects indicate statements for which they would be willing to take an oath of validity the error rate is around 5 to 10 per cent.

Thus to summarize early research it seems as if errors of testimony are almost unavoidable and that while interrogative measures are excellent means of filling out gaps in spontaneous report they have their dangers. They lead witnesses, especially children and unsophisticated adults, into false depositions. Falsification can be reduced but not completely eradicated by (1) asking for sworn statements, (2) obtaining the testimony as soon after the event as possible, (3) confining the testimony to that given in a spontaneous report and in answer to questions which are framed with as little suggestibility as possible. The conclusions of this early research would seem to be that if law enforcement agencies wish to minimize recall and statement error they should minimize the number and specificity of questions to be asked of the respondent. They should use only a small number of very broad open-ended questions whenever possible, and when a specific question is necessary a multi-choice procedure ought to be employed. However, closer inspection of the old results cast several doubts on these implications. The use of semi-structured or very structured questioning procedures can result in only a small increase in the amount of error obtained while at the same time significantly increasing the amount of material covered by testimony. The earlier findings of large increases in reported error resulting from the employment of specific questions can be explained by the failure to distinguish between the type of question asked and the difficulty of the information being sought (Marquis *et al.*, 1972). Marshall (1966) examined this possibility by looking at the effect of questioning on the accuracy of reporting three items. Specific questions increased the amount of testimony error for two items. These items were held to be difficult in the sense that they were seldom mentioned spontaneously in narrative testimony. An item which was reported by most people initially was answered correctly in response to specific questions.

Thus the possibility exists that it is not the form of the question itself which produces the inaccurate memory but rather the difficulty of the material being remembered. Therefore recent research has used a more intensive approach to the simple questions of whether narrative or interrogative approaches are better for eliciting accurate memory. Progressively experimentation has become multivalent and parametric rather than bivalent, i.e. different aspects of a number of factors have been investigated at one time, rather than merely looking at two aspects of one factor. A good example of this multi-variable approach is the study by Marquis *et al.* (1972). They at one and the same time sought to compare the accuracy and completeness of testimony under supportive and challenging atmospheres: to determine whether specific or more general questions were productive of greater accuracy; to see whether leading or non-leading questions influenced accuracy; and lastly they examined the interactive effect of these various factors. One hundred and fifty-one adults were presented with a one minute fifty-five second film and were then asked to give a free report of what they could remember and, following this, all subjects were allocated to one of eight interrogative conditions. Thus basically they had a narrative-interrogative format (as in earlier research). The film began with two boys throwing a ball around. The camera then panned from them over to a large building and parking lot, and stopped at the entrance to a supermarket where several people were emerging. In particular a man and a woman emerged, deep in discussion. The man then left the woman to fetch something he had forgotten, while the woman continued walking. She was then struck by a car leaving the parking lot. She lost her grip on her provisions and they fell to the ground. The driver got out of the car and said to her, 'Do you never watch where you are going?' at which point the 'victim' rose from the pavement and swore at him. Her companion came back, running and shouting, and a scuffle ensued between the two men. The companion was pushed to the ground and spilt his packages. The boys, who were earlier seen playing football, appeared, asked what happened and restrained the men. One of the boys then ran off towards the supermarket entrance to call the police. There were 884 scorable facts in the film. From these the authors selected a representative sample for specific questioning. Three broad types of possible question were generated: (1) legal relevance, (2) specific content (referring to persons, actions, sounds, objects, etc.), and (3) differentially salient questions (i.e. the more a pretest group of subjects mentioned an item the greater that item's saliency rating). This was used to assess the ease or difficulty of the item. Accuracy and completeness scores were computed for the types of question probed.

Errors were also scored and the number of correct items plus the number of error items constituted the number of items mentioned.

A number of the general findings are interesting. (1) Witnesses who were challenged by the questioner ('challenging atmosphere') were slightly more likely to think that the questioners wanted biased answers. (2) Those who were asked leading questions were more likely to expect that the questioner wanted them to distort their testimony. (3) In terms of the effect of the different types of questions greatest accuracy was found under free report, least accurate testimony being found under leading question conditions. (4) The type of atmosphere had little effect on accuracy or completeness of testimony. As question specificity increased there was an increase in the amount of material covered in testimony. Accuracy was highest for free report, next highest for the two open-ended interviews, and slightly lower for the interrogations using specific questions and forced choice answers. The effect of type of question on completeness index scores was very great and in the opposite direction. Large gains in completeness were accompanied by only small decreases in accuracy. The main effect, however, of the type of question on accuracy was mediated by item difficulty, such that the question type effect was greatest for difficult-to-remember items and weakest for easy material. Thus for free report, accuracy is high for both easy and difficult items but for structured questions (e.g. leading) accuracy is high for easy items but very low (about 50 per cent, chance level) for difficult items. Thus the conclusion from the earlier research on eyewitness testimony may need some qualification: structured questions introduce greater amounts of error but only for difficult items. Leading questions for difficult items produce much greater completeness than non-structured questions. For difficult items interviews which produced more data also resulted in increasing amounts of invalid data. For easy items more data did not mean more errors. The suggestion in this research then is that law enforcement agencies ought to be aware of the trade-off between accuracy and completeness which is a function of both the degree of specificity of the question and the difficulty of the to-be-recalled information. They should also consider using non-interview methods of collecting data about phenomena which are difficult for respondents to recall since these data are likely to be grossly inaccurate under structured questioning.

This research by Marquis *et al.* is, on the one hand, adding complexity which may eventually produce greater validity of data which could be used in non-laboratory situations and, on the other hand, is approximating real-life situations of crime episodes and police follow-ups. But there is still much further to go: one piece of research which goes some way towards experimentally manipulating customary police procedures is one by Alper, Buckhout, Chern, Harwood and Slomovits (1976). They compared reports by individuals and by those individuals acting together. The rationale for this experiment was that police are concerned to outline a coherent set of facts to explain all of the events under consideration in order to facilitate a 'search and find' procedure, or to prepare a case for the prosecution. To this end any one witness may fail to provide sufficient data either through poor attention, faulty perception or inadequate memory. Thus the natural remedy is to elicit a composite picture from the entire group of witnesses. The possible advantages of group recall over individual recall are fairly obvious – the greater overall detail, possible consensus, and screening out of irrelevancies. There is also the belief that two heads are better than one. In areas outside the psychology of visual memory it does seem as if groups do out-perform individuals, at least in some situations, for example, Hall, Mouton and Blake (1963) showed decisions reached in groups are superior to decisions based on the statistical pooling of individual judgments.

This book has been concerned to argue that individual recall or recognition in simulated reality experiments is poor, explicable on grounds of attention, perception, memory, stress, 'set' and environmental factors. Thus it is no surprise that the Warren Commission Report (1964) stressed composite descriptions and the accumulation of individual reports. However, other parts of this book have also hinted that reliance on consensual validation of uncheckable prior perceptions may be a dangerous business. Research on group dynamics in simple perceptual experiments would certainly suggest that this is possible (e.g. Sherrif and Asch on group conformity). Conformity is a fundamental insight in psychology which has crucial implications for eyewitness testimony. Alper *et al.* therefore set out to see if a group of witnesses to a simulated crime would be more accurate or less accurate in their collective recall than the recall achieved by averaging their individual testimonies.

One hundred and twenty-nine subjects witnessed an incident in a classroom which involved a student coming to the lecture and asking if he could look for a book he had left during the previous class. In the middle of his search the 'criminal' grabbed a student's pocket-book and ran from the classroom. The person whose pocket-book had been stolen ran out in hot pursuit, screaming as he went. After being informed that the incident had been staged, the witnesses were presented with a question-naire which asked for information on the incident, the descrip-tion of the criminal, and the witnesses' own relationship to the incident. During this phase of the experiment the witnesses were not allowed to consult one another. When the questionnaire had been completed, the subjects were then divided into four groups, and filled out the questionnaire again, this time as a group. It was stressed that only one answer to each individual question was permissible at this stage. The results were rather clear cut. Group consensus descriptions were more complete than averaged individual descriptions, with groups making on average 5.5 per cent errors of omission as compared with an average of 10 per cent errors for individuals. However, completeness was obtained at the cost of increased inaccuracy with groups obtaining 40 per cent more errors of commission than individuals. Group reports were more accurate in terms of estimation of the duration of the incident. While the actual time of the incident was 14 seconds, group estimates were 19.38 seconds and the individuals' average was 37.93 seconds. Groups underestimated weight by approxi-mately 10 lbs, individuals by approximately 5 lbs. Groups underestimated height while individuals overestimated.

Thus while groups produce greater completeness this may be a function of group conformity rather than composite memory. Group interaction may pressure witnesses into offering inferences rather than perceptions, or even into prefabrication. Studies in our own department (Clifford and Hollin, in prep.) support these suggestions. The study by Alper *et al.* can be criticized on a number of counts but chiefly because individual and group data are confounded with time since perceiving the event. One study which gets over this problem by using independent groups, i.e. by having one group discuss the incident and another, separate group not discuss it, but having both groups recall individually at the same delay since seeing the events, is one by Rupp, Warmbrand, Karash and Buckhout (1976). They showed that the interaction group produced a mean increase in the completeness of the description but no effect was found on recognition performance (a line-up). Interestingly, however, the discussion led some witnesses to change their descriptions to fit the available but innocent participants in the line-up.

Alper *et al.* concluded that group discussion with witnesses is an ill-advised procedure that may double the effort of the investigator and compound the error from both the legal and the perceptual point of view. This is a sound conclusion to draw but, unfortunately, in a real-life incident the group discussion occurs long before the police ever get to the scene. If one watches an incident – criminal or otherwise – a clear behaviour pattern emerges. Initially there is a 'freezing' then there is a 'mad panic' in which everyone wants to project their perception and understanding of the incident onto everyone else. Thus the possible detrimental nature of 'group discussion' operates even before the police can prevent it. What we must try and do is accept that it happens and try and explicate the mechanisms which are operative, and the implications for testimony and person identification. This we are doing at the North East London Polytechnic in a series of experiments carried out by the first author and Clive Hollin. While our first experiment was carried out before the Alper *et al.* study was published the results are very similar, but go beyond them in showing that if 'leaders' emerge in a group of witnesses the 'followers' will alter their testimony in line with the leaders' assertions even when the leaders are in error. This can give the illusion of certainty and consensus in a number of observers to a criminal incident, but in the laboratory, where objective truth can be checked, gross errors can be shown quite clearly to occur. Although there is strength in numbers there is, as Glanville Williams has pointed out, no real safety.

7 Individual and group differences in person recognition

The Devlin Report argued that there was no way in which we could distinguish between a valid testimony and an invalid one. This may be true, and may be in principle insoluble, but what can be done is to investigate groups or categories of potential witnesses in order to be able to give advice on whether special weight ought to be accorded to specifiable groups as such. This chapter will examine some factors which could explain and hopefully predict eyewitness ability.

AGE

When one compares the performance of younger and older people on a very wide range of intellectual tasks one normally finds that the older person performs better, provided that they are not too old. Since memory and perception are important determinants of intellectual functioning this same superiority of adults over younger children should still hold in identification. In tests of recognition memory for previously seen faces this superiority has been observed: Ellis, Shepherd and Bruce (1973) tested 12- and 17-year-old subjects and found the latter group to be much better at recognizing faces of young adults. One study, which at first sight appears to deny this relationship, is one by Cross, Cross and Daly (1971) where they looked for an improvement in face recognition with age but failed to find it in subjects aged 7, 12 or 17 years and adults. This surprising finding however was corrected by making use of the distinction we have already made – the distinction between 'false positive' and 'true positive' identification. Cross *et al.* found that the younger the children the more frequent was the error. That is, the younger subjects were guessing more often than were the older subjects, and thus by chance they were right more often. When a technique of calculation (d'), which gets over the problem of 'false positives', was applied to all the data the ranking of recognition performance from worst to best was 7, 12, 17 years and then adults.

When one ensures that the younger children's readiness to say that they had seen a face previously, when in fact they had not, is taken into account the ordering of superiority from younger to older is confirmed. The reasons for this ordering are numerous. One obvious explanation is in terms of familiarity. The older you are the more faces you have seen, and thus the more familiar you are with faces as such. That this is not the complete, nor the best, explanation (if it is an explanation at all) is indicated by the findings of Goldstein and Chance (1964) who failed to show that young children are better at recognizing faces drawn from their own age group, which they would be more familiar with, than faces drawn from a different age group.

A prediction from general cognitive development, character-ized as a process of increasingly sophisticated ways of perceiving, processing, storing, manipulating and retrieving material, would suggest the ordering from younger to older found in the above studies. As such the argument is that memorial performance with seen faces is merely one aspect of the more general facility older subjects have in handling all types of information.

Now while this ordering from younger to older is well pre-dicted from general cognitive psychology there is one line of research, from experimental psychology, which would not pre-dict such an order: it is to this line of research we now turn.

EIDETIC IMAGERY

Eidetic imagery is more widely, but mistakenly, known as 'photographic memory'. Eidetic imagery has been defined by Landauer (1972) as 'the ability to retain an accurate, detailed visual image of a complex scene or pattern' and by Kagan and Havemann (1972) as 'the ability, possessed by a minority of people, to "see" an image that is an exact copy of the original sensory experience'. The important point to emphasize here is that 'the minority of people' who possess eidetic imagery are children. The original belief was that children had such powers; adults did not. For the case of person recognition and identification this would seem to have crucial implications because if children have eidetic imagery, characterized by clarity, persistence and vividness, whilst an adult only has 'ordinary' visual imagery which is characterized as being 'incomplete and usually unstable' (Richardson, 1969), then children ought to be much more reliable witnesses.

What is the reality? The phenomenon of eidetic imagery was discovered over a century ago, and the work up to 1976 has been reviewed, in chronological order, by Allport (1924), Jaensch (1930), Kluver (1932), Haber (1969), Richardson (1969) and Gray and Gummerman (1975). The existence of eidetic imagery has been detected by two chief methods: (1) a subjective report technique called picture description, and (2) an objective method called the superimposition method. The picture description method is very simple procedurally. The subject sits in front of a screen or easel upon which a picture is projected or rested, and after a certain time the projected image or photograph is removed and the subject is asked to give a verbal description of the now absent picture. The criteria whereby one decides whether eidetic imagery is present or not in the subject are numerous and not at all well articulated. Eidetic imagery is assumed to be present if the person reports the presence of vivid imagery and if they report that they still 'see' the picture. Confidence is another measure, plus the use of the present tense ('I see' rather than 'I saw'). Jaensch has argued that the accuracy and the extensiveness of the report are crucial to the deduction of eidetic imagery presence. However, Leask, Haber and Haber (1969) reported little correlation between accuracy and the other indicators of eidetic ability. Thus Haber (1969) concluded that accuracy was not a reliable criterion. If, however, eidetikers have 'extended perceptual experiences' then they ought to be remarkably accurate, thus Haber's position seems odd. Another interesting index of whether a person has eidetic imagery is the presence of eye movements. The argument, broadly stated, is that if the eidetiker projects the image 'out there' then that image ought to be scanned in the same way as when a person is asked to describe a picture which he is looking at directly.

Given that these indices, either separately or in combination, provide some reliability then it becomes legitimate to look at other questions which have potential relevance to eyewitness reliability. One such question is how frequent in the population is the ability found and who has it? Kluver (1931) has reported rates as low as 0 per cent and as high as 100 per cent. These wildly fluctuating estimates obviously stem from the poor use of common measuring instruments or criteria. From the new interest in the phenomenon which began in about 1960 much greater consistency in measurement has been seen and thus a more stable body of findings has emerged. The range is now seen to be from 0 per cent (e.g. Traxel, 1962), with normal children to 11 per cent by Furst, Fuld and Pancoe (1974), also with normal children. Gummerman, Gray and Wilson (1972) produced evidence of 0 per cent in normal adults.

Of direct relevance to this book is the type of material which has been used to test for eidetic imagery. Jaensch noted that eidetic imagery was difficult to elicit unless the stimulus picture contained interesting material. Further, the parts of the picture had to have some inner connection or structure that was appropriate to 'the laws of imagination' (Jaensch, 1930). This fact admits of two possible explanations: either the material had to be interesting to keep the person motivated and attentive, or meaningful structured material has greater contact with stored schemata and therefore allows greater constructive facility (e.g. Neisser, 1967). The importance of these opposing interpretations is that they hit at the very question of whether eidetic imagery is a perceptual facility separate from memory (seen as organized stocks of past experience), or whether it is merely a form of visual imagery intimately connected with such memory. If eidetic imagery is a pure perceptual phenomenon unrelated to memory schemata then it should make no difference whether the parts of the stimulus are integrated into a meaningful whole or not because all parts will be equally well registered visually and thus capable of being projected as an eidetic image. If, however, eidetic imagery stems from interpretation of input by existing schemata then the prediction would be that only if the input 'matches' existing schemata (which are organized) will eidetic imagery be possible. That is, a disorganized and un-structured input should not give rise to eidetic imagery. The findings of Jaensch (1930) can be cited as evidence for the latter view. He presented a scene, constructed by putting together items cut from other scenes and which therefore lacked internal coherence, and failed to elicit eidetic imagery in subjects pre-viously rated as eidetic. This finding has very close parallels with studies quoted in other parts of this book, especially in Chapter 2 where schema-driven perceptions were discussed.

Under the heading of eidetic research a most informative study is one by Leask *et al.* (1969) who presented a 'rogues' gallery' of 25 cartoon faces arranged in a 5 x 5 display, and found that eidetic imagery was not forthcoming. Leask *et al.* conclu-ded that the display lacked cohesiveness, therefore rendering the stimulus very difficult, and thus disrupted the eidetic process. We can then ask if the eidetic process would also be disrupted by one face presented in motion as happens at the scene of a crime.

Over and above the question of who exhibits eidetic imagery and what types of situation evoke it, a most crucial question for us is just how accurate is an eidetiker, if such a person exists? To recap, the argument is that certain people have photographic memories; it is children who have such abilities; and this ability is characterized by its fidelity to the actual input. It is a short step from these premises to the assertion that therefore children will make excellent witnesses. However, even in persons who exhibit eidetic imagery accuracy is far from perfect. High accuracy was shown in the study by Haber and Haber (1964) where eidetikers were sufficiently accurate to describe the number of feathers worn by each of ten pictured Indians. Low accuracy has also been reported however, by among others, Gummerman *et al.* (1972) and Meenes and Morton (1936).

Another question which law enforcement agencies would want clarified is how long does the eidetic image last. Gray and Gummerman (1975) suggest that the typical range is 30–40 seconds, but that it could be as long as 3–5 minutes, or more. In fact one of the very few adult eidetikers (Elizabeth), when tested under the objective approach (to be discussed below), showed no fading of the most complex random dot patterns after twenty-four hours (Stromeyer, 1970; Stromeyer and Psotka, 1970). However, the general proposition is that there are very large differences both within and between subjects in their ability to retain an image. Leask *et al.* (1969) suggested that once an image has faded it could not be fetched back. From this it would seem that even if children did exhibit eidetic imagery it would not be of any great help in identification, given the long delays in most actual criminal cases between the witness observing the criminal and being asked to attend an identification parade. It could however be of use in giving descriptions of a seen criminal if statements were taken immediately after the crime, but this all depends on the reality of the concept of eidetic imagery.

From what has been said above it can be seen that the evidence which comes from the subjective report method of picture description is at best tentative and at worst fairly negative in terms of the reality of a special ability called eidetic imagery. Is the evidence any stronger from the more objective approach of superimposition?

The superimposition method basically involves asking the subject to 'project' his image onto a screen at the same time as the experimenter is projecting a different scene onto the same screen. The argument is that if the subject is in fact 'projecting' an eidetic image this will fuse with the actual image that the experimenter is presenting and any report by the eidetiker should contain elements of this fused stimulus. That is, the person will report seeing objects or details which are neither present in the original stimulus which occasioned the eidetic image nor the image which the experimenter is currently projecting, but only in the fused composite of the two. The initial problem with such fusion studies was that the fusion could be predicted from viewing the two stimuli separately. Fortunately later studies have utilized material in which such prediction of the fusion is not possible. One of these studies was conducted by Leask *et al.* (1969) who presented a stimulus such that the composite (fusion) was a schematic face. Four out of twenty-three eidetikers were able to identify the composite.

While the technique of superimposition has the potentiality of objectivity the findings are somewhat conflicting, and the safest conclusion would seem to be one along the lines of Gray and Gummerman (1975), that the reality of eidetic imagery has not been established. Before this is uncritically accepted, however, Gray and Gummerman argue that the stimuli used in fusion studies of necessity had to be complex, but we have shown above that eidetic imagery is most likely to occur with simple material of a meaningful nature. Another possibility is that fusion studies require stereoscopic skills which may not yet have developed in children, and we have seen that if eidetic ability does exist then almost certainly it is to be found in children.

What has been stressed throughout this section is not that rather spectacular feats of visual memory never occur, nor that the potential of such abilities should not be studied within an applied psychology of person identification, rather we are denying that such ability is something distinct from visual memory in general, and that it is something unique to children. The position taken here is that argued by Marsh and Abbot (1945) and later by Gray and Gummerman (1975) in which only one imagery system is postulated and that it is cognitive rather than perceptual. As support for this thesis it can be shown that (a) structural material is better remembered than unstructured material, (b) verbal rehearsal of visual material presented to evoke eidetic imagery prevents such eidetic imagery from being produced, (c) focusing attention on particular aspects of an eidetic image can cause those aspects to disappear, (d) the parts of an eidetic image fade in a principled way, not at random, (e) the facts of eidetic imagery overlap with the facts of visual imagery such that both are positively coloured, both are reported confidently, eye movements do not correlate in a one-to-one fashion with either eidetic or visual imagery, and lastly both high and low accuracy has been recorded under both types of imagery.

Thus the common sense belief that young children are better witnesses than adults because of their eidetic imagery is fallacious. Eidetic imagery is a very infrequent phenomenon and where it does exist it merely refers to a highly efficient functioning of the perceptual-memorial-cognitive system, eidetic imagery simply being the 'good' end of the visual imagery system. As such then the experimental line of evidence which suggested that children should be better than adults in a recognition situation, in contrast to the developmental argument outlined at the end of the previous section on age, has not been substantiated. The working hypothesis that the older the witness, up to a point, the better or more reliable the testimony or recognition therefore still holds. Not only does it hold but it is strengthened by · other research.

INDIVIDUAL DIFFERENCES IN TERMS OF SUGGESTIBILITY

There are two oppposing views here. One says that a adults develop so their perception becomes much more conditioned by their existing stocks of knowledge. Thus the older one is the more one is liable to interpret what one sees rather than store it literally. On this view children should be better witnesses. The other, social, psychological view however is that person recognition is in real life a social interaction situation (Clifford, 1975) and the possibility exists that wherever there are interactive contacts suggestibility and biasing can come into play. Now this argument makes the same prediction as the cognitive development hypotheses, viz. that children will be poorer witnesses, because they are more susceptible to suggestion.

We saw in Chapter 6 on recall under questioning that Stern estimated that 7-year-olds are misled by 50 per cent of questions, as contrasted with 18-year-olds who are misled by only 20 per cent. Otis (1924) shows clearly that children are more open to suggestion than adults. Gray and Gummerman (1975) also use this argument to explain the fact that eidetic imagery is regarded as a childhood phenomenon. Children may have no greater visual imagery than adults but because of greater suggestibility they may be more open to task demands in the laboratory and suggestive questions in the real-life situation of person and event recall under police questioning. Sheehan and Neisser (1969) show clearly that visual perceptions can be influenced markedly by minor details of experimental procedure. Again, in terms of eidetic imagery, the practice sessions, which precede the study phase of the experiment, and which are employed to establish willingness to respond, clearly are a source of suggestion for the statement that eidetic images are located 'out there' (Allport, 1928; Kluver, 1932; Traxel, 1962).

If suggestion can be shown to be a crucial factor in eliciting eidetic images how much more likely is it in real life where the children are asked for recall or recognition of a fast-moving visual event or object?

INDIVIDUAL DIFFERENCES IN IMAGERY ABILITY

When one reads the law journals or popular press one frequently comes across the phrase 'visual memory image' applied to perception and memory, or the remembering of a scene. The implicit assumption seems to be that everyone possesses this to the same extent and it thus becomes simply a case of reading off from this image when one attends an identification parade or tries to help the police in the reconstruction of a criminal incident. Such is not the case; just as there are tall or short people, fat or thin people, so there are good visualizers and poor visualizers. The reasons for this are many and diverse and will not be examined here. Richardson (1969) talks of habitual visualizers and habitual verbalizers. It would, however, be totally wrong to think of the entire population as divided into these two mutually exclusive types. Grey Walter (1953) estimated the incidence of 'types' in an unselected population as being 15 per cent habitual visualizers, 15 per cent habitual verbalizers, and the remaining 70 per cent being able to utilize whichever of the two modes was demanded by the task, or by personal preference. Harris and Haber (1963) looked at the ways in which 77 subjects encoded a visual stimulus: 75 of the 77 subjects coded in terms of verbal form because rehearsal was encouraged and it is difficult to rehearse a visual trace. Bartlett (1932) noted that the same subjects used the same encoding medium (verbal or visual) irrespective of the type of material presented. As Richardson (1969) and McKellar (1972) also suggest, while the ability to generate and employ imagery varies across people the potential to do so is universal. Marks (1972) says, 'given appropriate and optimal conditions of training and performance it is likely that all persons could utilize imagery-encoded information.'

Given then that we can delineate two broad types of persons – the habitual visualizer and the habitual verbalizer – what is the significance of this for person recognition? The answer is that the ability to form images may facilitate memory for a seen face. No work, to the present authors' knowledge, has looked at this but when good visualizers and poor visualizers have been tested on ability to recall or recognize previously seen objects and events, the high visualizer has always produced better performance. However, let us look first at the negative evidence. Bartlett (1932) argued that imagery was a hindrance. He argued that the appearance of a visual image was followed by an increase of confidence entirely out of proportion with any objective accuracy. Generally speaking, Bartlett also found that imagery interfered with memory for order or sequence information. The problem, however, with all the early work, which was predominantly negative concerning the function of imagery, was that they had no objective measure of whether imagery had in fact taken place, and also, it was conducted on verbal material. More recent studies clearly demonstrate that imagery can play a powerful role in memory. One such series of studies by Sheehan (1966, 1967; Sheehan and Neisser, 1969) shows clearly that imagery is a useful source of information in the performance of certain cognitive tasks. Broadly speaking, the main findings of the various studies are that accuracy of recall is correlated with vividness of imagery ratings, that the encoding strategies of poor and vivid imagers differ, and third, that the relationship between imagery and stimulus complexity is not simple.

A second series of experiments which looked at individual differences (high and low visualizers) in terms of accuracy of recall of visually presented pictures is that by Marks (1972). Marks used a picture memory task in conjunction with a vividness of visual imagery questionnaire (VVIQ). The picture memory task employed pictorial and coloured stimuli, of which half were sets of fifteen unrelated objects and the other half photographs of scenes (e.g. a Venice canal, a New York street, a group of bathers, a market place, a Turkish pavement scene). The subjects were allowed to observe the projected stimuli for twenty seconds, and were then prevented from rehearsing for forty seconds, and were eventually given questions of the following type: 'What colour was the woman's hat – yellow and red, white and red, or yellow and white?' Subjects chose one answer from the three alternatives provided. Marks (1972) was interested in the number of incorrect answers. The good visualizers performed much better than the poor visualizers and the good female visualizers performed better than did the good male visualizers. A replicative refinement was performed of this experiment and again the same two results appeared, but even more strongly. Poor visualizers made 36 per cent more errors than good visualizers. Further, greater accuracy went with greater vividness of imagery. Marks concludes that these studies show, along with Sheehan (1966), that people who report (objectively verified) vivid visual imagery can produce more accurate recall of pictorial material than those who report poor visual imagery.

Before we conclude this section it ought to be pointed out that the studies by Sheehan and by Marks investigated literal imagery which is defined as that type of imagery which is used when a person is asked to remember a stimulus pattern. Other types of imagery exist, which could have direct relevance to person recognition. It is possible that on seeing a criminal a witness will label him and from this label generate an image unconsciously. This associative imagery could greatly hinder accurate description or recognition of the criminal at some later date.

SEX DIFFERENCES

The general finding is that females are better than males at recognizing faces they have previously seen. This general finding, however, needs qualification. One needs to distinguish between real-life and laboratory findings; one also needs to specify the sex of the observers and the observed face; and, third, one has to be aware of whether real life, photographed or schematic faces are being used as the testing material.

Given these three qualifications the research findings are fairly clear. McKelvie (1972) found no sex differences in recognition of schematic faces, and Howells (1938) also found no difference with photographs. These two studies, however, are somewhat against the tide because Goldstein and Chance (1971) did find a difference between men and women observers when they presented photographs of faces, snowflakes and inkblots for later recognition. The females were better than males, but only for faces. It should be noted that only female faces were presented as stimuli. Cross, Cross and Daly (1971) failed to show an overall female superiority with both male and female photographs as stimuli. However, the female observers performed significantly better than male observers on female faces, with the male observers being equally good on the male and female faces. Witryol and Kaess (1957) did show women to be superior overall compared to men but also found that male observers were better with male faces and female observers were better with female faces. In a similar way Ellis, Shepherd and Bruce (1973) found that while there was no significant difference between male and female observers for male faces, there was a significant difference for female faces, with women performing better. Studies by both McCall, Mazanec, Erikson and Smith (1974), and Mazanec and McCall (1975) show female superiority in observational accuracy on a number of tests, but again they are concerned to stress the 'same sex effect', i.e. that females do better with female stimuli than with male stimuli persons.

Referring back to the imagery section of this chapter, it should be remembered that Marks (1972) found a female superiority in both his studies where the observers were asked to recall details of scenes and haphazard collections of objects. In contrast to this study we will show below that Schill (1966) found no sex differences in an incidental memory for faces task, which could, however, be accounted for by personality differences cutting across the sex factor.

How can the weight of evidence in favour of women be explained? A number of possibilities exist. Cross *et al.* and Ellis *et al.* explained their findings of female superiority by the greater exposure of females to female faces in magazines and cosmetic literature, and thus the increased opportunity to learn to encode features of faces. There is also evidence that women may be more socially attentive (e.g. Exline, 1963; Witryol and Kaess, 1957). A third possible explanation is that of motivation (Smith, 1966), personality differences and cognitive style, which we will be reviewing next, (e.g. Bruner, Goodnow and Austin, 1956; Garai and Scheinfeld, 1968). Women are more field-dependent than men and field-dependence correlates positively with memory for faces (Messick and Damarin, 1964). A fourth explanation of female superiority may have an ontogenetic component. Fagan (1972) showed that 5- to 6-month-old girls appear to have better memory for photographs of faces than their male counterparts. However, this cannot be a perceptual maturity because Hutt (1972) reviewed a large amount of evidence which showed that infant boys exhibit more interest in visual patterns than do girls. The answer may lie (e.g. Ellis, 1975) in the fact that girls learn to associate sounds with faces earlier than boys, and Hutt indicates that girls are more responsive than boys to sounds. This whole ontogenetic argument is, however, weakened by the fact that Fagan (1973, 1976) failed to replicate his previous sex difference findings, although Haaf and Brown (1976) did note a complex sex effect in 15-week-old infants observing facial and non-facial stimuli which could vary in degree of complexity – females fixating longer than males at the more complex levels of facial stimuli. Until now sex difference findings have been drawn from studies on schematic and photographic faces. Does female superiority also hold in real-life or simulated crime studies? It appears that it does not. Kuehn (1974) showed that female victims are poorer at giving complete descriptions of assailants, whereas Bahrick, Bahrick and Wittlinger (1975) indicate that in non-emotionally charged atmospheres female superiority does reassert itself in recognition and recall of people who have been interacted with. Research carried out at North East London Polytechnic (Clifford and Scott, in press) has shown that when a non-violent episode is viewed for later recollection female witnesses are better than males, but when a violent episode is viewed, later recall by males is superior to that of females. Thus females were found to perform poorly under stressful conditions, a finding that supports Kuehn's tabulation of real-life police-elicited recalls from male and female victims.

While an obvious point, we feel that it ought to be stressed that male-female difference findings are based on average differences, and variability must be expected. Two males on the same task can differ much more than a male and a female on that task, at a specific time. But, generally speaking, females are better at recognizing previously seen faces in non-emotive situations. Under stressful viewing conditions males may make the better type of witness.

COGNITIVE STYLE

Kogan (1970) has defined cognitive style as an individual's mode of perceiving, remembering and thinking, or as his characteristic ways of 'apprehending, storing, transforming and utilizing information'. Police officers and courts of law are concerned with the abilities of witnesses, but judgments as to the validity of such testimony can be crucially informed by knowledge of the mode or manner of individual information processing styles. While the literature on cognitive style has proliferated since the 1960s, as shown by the interchangeability of such terms as 'cognitive control principles', 'cognitive strategies', and 'modes of information processing' the area has been rendered tractable by Messick (1970) who lists nine distinguishable processing styles. He argues that individuals can be shown to differ along the dimension of field-dependence/field-independence; in terms of attention deployment (scanning); in breadth of categorization; in conceptual styles; along the continuum of cognitive complexity-cognitive simplicity; reflective-impulsive; levelling-sharpening; constricted or flexible control; and finally tolerance of ambiguity. To this list of nine cognitive styles, Kogan (1970) adds a tenth – risk taking and cautiousness. Only those cognitive styles which have direct relevance to person identification in particular, and eyewitnesses in general, will be discussed here.

Field-independence refers to a way of perceiving which entails a tendency to experience items as discrete and separable from the background factors in which they are embedded. Basically in the perceptual realm, field-independence reflects the ability to focus attention of the important parts of a scene and to avoid the confusing influence of the embedding context. Field-dependence is the converse of the above.

As a result of these different styles of perception it has frequently been argued (Witkin, Dyk, Faterson, Goodenough and Karp, 1974), that while field-independent subjects are better at performing cognitive tasks, the field-dependent person is better at socially relevant activities and, indeed, Fitzgibbons, Goldberg and Eagle (1965) showed that field-dependent subjects were better than field-independent subjects at remembering socially orientated words. Most suggestively in the field of facial memory, Messick and Damarin (1964) indicated the possibility of predicting recognition performance from knowledge of differences between people in field-dependence and field-independence. On the basis of two studies, one of which showed that field-dependent subjects could recognize cut out features from their own faces better than could field-independent subjects (De Varis, unpublished), and the second of which indicated that field-dependent Air Force officers were better than field-independent officers at correctly recognizing photographs of people who had been living in close proximity with them (Crutchfield, Woodworth and Albrecht, 1958), Messick and Damarin predicted that field-dependent subjects ought to remember seen photographed faces better than field-independent subjects under disguised memory conditions (i.e. in incidental memory situations). In their experiment subjects were presented with photographs of ten types of person and were then asked to rate each presented person for age and to indicate if any looked like some individual who had been encountered previously in the observers' everyday lives. The types of person portrayed were teenagers, youthful, middle-aged and elderly men, a similar four-fold set of females, and in addition groups of middle-aged men selected to typify 'strength' and 'weakness'. Various poses were used such as serious or smiling. The main finding was that field-dependent subjects produced better recognition than field independent subjects. Interestingly in terms of the thesis developed throughout this book, 42 per cent of subjects wrongly identified a never before seen face as having been previously presented. It seems possible that because field-dependent subjects have a high need for satisfaction of social drives they have developed skills of processing and storing faces in order to 'read' the social situation.

It is unfortunate that in this study Messick and Damarin did not have equal numbers of males and females because research indicates that females are better than males at recognizing faces, and that females are more field-dependent than males (e.g. Witkin, Dyk, Faterson, Goodenough and Karp, 1962). If this had been done we could have achieved some indication of the relative effects of sex and personality in person recognition. Messick and Damarin also showed that narrow categorizers were relatively better than broad categorizers in recognition of the presented faces. This superiority may be due to learned skills of perception and classification which eventuate in better registration of facial features, finer sensitivity to small differences in facial configuration and, more speculatively, different guessing strategies. One interesting non-predicted finding was the possibility of a subject's affective response to a face. To judge a face favourably may result in increased and closer attention to the features, attributes and expressions that serve to individualize that face. The avoidance of physical contact with 'undesirables' may be mirrored in the avoidance of perceptual contact and attention to details of the faces of such persons, thus decreasing eventual recognition and recall performance.

The implication of the above studies seems to be that field-dependent observers would be better eyewitnesses than field-independent observers, other things being equal. There is, however, another possible explanation of field-dependents' superiority and that is that they may be more prone to inter-personal accommodation, and less able to resist social pressure (e.g. Linton, 1955). Wallach, Kogan and Burt (1967) compared field-dependent and field-independent subjects in discussion groups and found that field-dependent subjects took less time to reach a consensus. In terms of the studies carried out by the first author at the North East London Polytechnic into conformity effects on eyewitness testimony this could suggest that field-dependent subjects would make poor witnesses because observers can agree in error.

Over and above this 'willingness to respond' on the part of the field-dependent subject, which could result in high levels of false recognition, there are a number of studies which suggest that, in fact, field-*independent* subjects would make the better witnesses. Observers rated as field-independent have been shown to be more accurate in recognition of photographed faces under both incidental learning conditions (Baker, 1967; Beijk-Docter and Elshout, 1969), and intentional learning conditions (Adcock and Webberley, 1971; Hoffman and Kagan, 1977). In the Hoffman and Kagan study however this superiority only held for males, field-independent females being non-significantly better than field-dependent females.

From these several studies it thus appears that the prediction of eyewitness reliability from knowledge of an observers field-dependence/field-independence status would not be easy. Future research will have to look closely at the sex of the witness and the nature of the witnessing situation. Also it will have to consider the relationship between performance on photographs of faces and performance with live targets. It is unfortunate that the only study to do this (Crutchfield *et al.*, 1958) was so fraught with problems of control that clear conclusions could not be drawn. Finally, the modifiability of witness behaviour must now be considered against the background of more general knowledge concerning field-dependence/field-independence.

Witkin *et al.* (1962) stressed that females were more field-dependent than males, and this would tie in with female superiority in terms of face recognition. Over and above sex differences it seems as if field-dependence/field-independence is fairly stable over the age range 8–24 years (Witkin, Goodenough and Karp, 1967) but there is a slight tendency to become more field-independent as one becomes older. Because field-dependence/field-independence in perception is merely one aspect of a more enduring personality 'type' remediation programmes would seem to have poor prognosis, short-term training not having been very successful (e.g. Elliot and McMichael, 1963).

Reflective and impulsive cognitive styles also have implications for person recognition. This 'style' or dimension refers to the willingness of people to pause and reflect upon the accuracy of their perceptions, hypotheses and solutions. Some people act upon their first hypothesis and pay little heed to correctness or appropriateness, and it seems that young children are more impulsive than older children. The generality of an impulsive or reflective manner seems quite wide, and Kogan (1970) says that it 'seems to be the case that in all tasks which have a response uncertainty aspect the distinction between fast and slow subjects can be shown'. Modifiability of this cognitive style has been shown (e.g. Debus, 1970; Nelson, 1968) but for our purposes, the reduction of error rates in perceptual tasks evidently requires specific training in scanning visual arrays. Given that the basic task in impulsive/reflective research involves matching a number of alternatives (only one of which is correct) to a standard, the similarity to identification parades is compelling and much more research needs to be carried out concerning this cognitive style factor within the context of the psychology of person recognition.

Levelling-sharpening is the one cognitive style which deals

specifically with individual differences in memory functioning. Levellers show a tendency to assimilate new perceptions to previously perceived and stored material. In contrast, sharpeners are able to keep memories of prior stimuli and current information separate. Gardner and Long (1960) showed that this cognitive style is fairly stable over a three year period, but that over and above this stability there may also be an increase in sharpening as one gets older (Gardner and Moriarty, 1968), at least between the ages of 9 to 13 years. Given that sharpeners would make the better witnesses, once again it can be seen that older children should be better witnesses than younger children. The applicability of this cognitive dimension is suggested by Holzman and Gardner (1960) who showed that children known to be sharpeners recalled more details of well known children's stories than did levellers.

Risk taking and cautiousness is the last 'style' we shall look at. Some individuals see risk as a value (e.g. Brown, 1965) and exhibit such risk taking as one aspect of a highly generalized motivational disposition. An identification parade represents a miniature decision-making situation in which the person is in possession of partial knowledge and thus risks must be taken. The disposition of individuals towards risk or caution will affect the decision to guess or not to guess.

The various cognitive styles discussed above can be seen to be fairly consistent and stable, and their generality across various tasks can be demonstrated. Of importance to the psychology of person identification is the fact that most of these styles are very easily assessed. In most cases one single test can indicate a person's standing along the relevant dimension. If law enforcement bodies wished to obtain some indication of a person's reliability as a witness this could quickly and efficiently be obtained. But only a suggestion as to the person's reliability could be achieved by such tests because the adequate perception, encoding, storing and retrieving of a crime or criminal is a multi-determined act which cannot be adequately or fully assessed by recourse to cognitive style alone. In terms of potential training programmes, it is still undecided whether cognitive styles are learned or innate, and thus, just how modifiable they are is not known. As Kogan (1970) points out, 'those cognitive styles which have the quality of a capacity are more resistant to modification than those styles which have the properties of a strategy.' If cognitive styles could be modified this would be a bonus, but at the moment what we can say is that a theoretical awareness of such modes of processing information is important for any real understanding of why witnesses make the errors they do, and why some witnesses are 'intrinsically' better than others. The hope is that eventually we can go beyond understanding to prediction, but this is for the future.

PERSONALITY DIFFERENCES

Need for Approval

A truism of everyday life is that each individual is unique. This uniqueness is encapsulated in the person's personality which Eysenck (1947) has defined as the 'sum total of the actual or potential behaviour patterns of the organism, as determined by heredity and environment'. However, human interaction is predicted upon a belief in consistency such that despite his uniqueness, every individual is to a certain extent predictable. This probabilistic approach to individuals and groups of individuals renders social life possible and scientific psychology tractable. Tractability is achieved by talking about dimensions or categories of personality and within these, 'traits' are used as fairly specific labels for groups of behaviour. One such trait is need-for-approval (n-App). Crowne and Marlow (1964) argued that a person who is characterized by high n-App has a low and vulnerable level of self-esteem. This becomes a motivational determinant of a socially desirable response set. The n-App person constantly seeks the approval of others as one means of bolstering his self-esteem.

This personality trait has implications for eyewitness reliability because a prediction from knowledge of the n-App literature is that such a person should be sensitive to inter-personal cues in social situations, and the face, *par excellence*, is the carrier of such cues. These predictions were put to the test by Schill (1966) who compared male and female, high and low n-App subjects on an incidental memory-for-faces task. The photographs used were the same as those used by Messick and Damarin which we discussed in the previous section above. Forty-two male and forty-two females were asked to estimate the age of each of the eighty persons shown in the photographs, but they were not told to expect a recognition test. Exposure duration was ten seconds, and ten minutes elapsed between initial presentation of the photographs and subsequent presentation for recognition, during which time all the subjects filled out a test sheet which rated them for high or low n-App. The recognition part of the experiment involved the presentation of twenty 'old' (previously shown) and twenty 'new' (not previously shown) photographs. Subjects were asked to state whether or not each photograph had been presented previously. High n-App subjects performed better than low n-App subjects, and there was no difference between male and female observers. Again, however, false-positives were problematic. It was found that high n-App subjects produced significantly more wrong identifications than did low n-App subjects. Again there was no sex difference. This last finding suggests that high n-App subjects, in their desire to gain approval, were willing to 'guess' that a face had been seen previously when in fact it had not. This has important implications for law enforcement and the execution of judicial process.

The general finding of more correct identification of faces by high n-App subjects would seem to reflect the fact that because these subjects are geared to protect self-esteem and to receive social reinforcements they have learned to attend more intensely to faces than low n-App subjects. This, however, cannot be substantiated in this study because fixation time was not recorded, but it does seem intuitively plausible. Like the study by Messick and Damarin an interesting finding emerged which may have implications for police forces. One condition in the experiment provided disapproval, during the initial perception of the faces, of high n-App subjects (the experimenter shook his head and said 'bad guess' as subjects judged the ages of the person photographed) and this produced a significant drop in correct recognition. Schill concludes that where self-esteem is threatened high n-App subjects may show a defensive, repressive strategy, whereby they actively cease to process the input. If it could be shown that disapproval also hinders retrieval then witnesses who are high or low on n-App would react differently to high or low status questioners, or nurturant and aggressive interrogators. In Chapter 2 it was shown that unpleasant situations could produce failure in retrieval when learning had been assured (see Kline, 1972, for a review).

Need for Affiliation

This is another 'trait' upon which individuals have been shown to differ. This trait has been defined by Murray (1938) as the need to 'draw near, to please and to win affection of' another social person. Thus the need for affiliation (n-Aff) is characterized by a desire to be with people in an affectionate and friendly relationship. The question then arises does n-Aff influence performance in ways which could have significance for person identification? One way in which it may relate is in an increased perceptual sensitivity to human faces in people high on n-Aff. This was put to the test by Atkinson and Walker (1955) who pointed out that motives can sensitize perception for motive-related stimuli. The theoretical rationale for their study was that faces are a class of stimuli related to affiliation. Ninety-three subjects were presented with eighty trials, each trial comprising a slide which had four objects displayed in the four possible quadrants, top, bottom, left and right. All stimuli were below recognition threshold (that is they were not able to be seen clearly), and the subjects were asked to indicate, for each trial, that quadrant which stood out the most or was the clearest. Unknown to the subjects, on each slide one quadrant contained a face, or a group of faces, the other three positions being filled with pictures of household objects. The placement of the face(s) and other objects was randomly allocated to the four quadrants for each trial. It was found that subjects high in n-Aff selected the face quadrant significantly more frequently than did subjects low in n-Aff. These findings can be taken as tentative support for the belief that a person's motives can sensitize his perceptual selection of motive-relevant stimuli; in the case of high n-Aff this would be faces. Thus a tentative speculation would be that high n-Aff subjects ought to make good witnesses.

Introverts and Extroverts

These terms were first used by Jung but have been given major explanatorv value by H. J. Eysenck. Broadly speaking, extroversion refers to the kind of behaviour which is out-going, or outwardly orientated. The person is highly aware of what is going on around him and he relates to outside objects and people. The introverted personality on the other hand is inward looking, orientation is towards self, and the understanding of one's own experiences.

H. J. Eysenck's work since about 1953 has been an attempt to elucidate the physiological determinants and concomitants of these two types of personality. The generally accepted position is that introverts are more aroused than extroverts. However, it is also possible that introverts and extroverts have the same amount of arousal but different optimal arousal levels, with the optimal arousal level of extroverts being higher than introverts. More recently M. W. Eysenck (1976) has argued that it is rather important to distinguish between arousal in the sense of a person's transient level of arousal (e.g. in the laboratory or at the scene of a crime), and arousal in the sense of a person's more enduring level of activation or arousal in everyday situations. A few seconds' consideration of stage fright and examination nerves should suggest to the reader that a high level of arousal can often prevent accurate memorization, or to put it more scientifically, can interfere with retrieval of stored information. This suggests the broad generalization that introverts should be poorer at memory tasks than extroverts, and generally speaking this is the case. Extroverts show better memory over short periods of time, but introverts are better at longer delays. Broadbent (1971) argues that under high arousal processing is focused on dominant sources of stimulation (i.e. important or salient features), at the expense of less dominant and unimportant features. M. W. Eysenck (1976) argues that the same process operates at output. He argues that high arousal biases the person's search process towards readily accessible, or functionally dominant, stored information (stereotypes?) more than is the case with lower levels of arousal.

Arousal can be increased either by external events or internal perceptions and this whole area of research would seem to have vital significance to the area of person identification seen as a four-stage process. These stages are perception at crime, storage, identification parades and identification. Much more research must be conducted here. Only a few rather dated research papers are available. Gilliland and Burke (1926) presented faces for immediate recall and found that extroverts were significantly better than introverts. Hunt (1928) found a correlation of +0.55 between extroversion and memory for names and faces (which was a subtest of a much larger test). Extroversion and introversion have also been linked with imagery ability. Gale, Morris, Lucas, and Richardson (1972) reported a significant correlation between performance on a version of the Betts Vividness of Imagery Scale and extroversion. Extroverts reported more vivid imagery than did introverts, and this relationship was supported by Morris and Gale (1974). As we have argued above, individual differences in vividness of imagery correlate with performance in memory tasks (e.g. Marks, 1972) and thus it is possible that the short-term superiority of extroverts is mediated by imagery coding. The problem here is that the rated amount of imagery evoked by separate words does not correlate with extroversion. The correlation of imagery evocation and introversion/extroversion is even more confused by the study of Huckabee (1974), who showed that it was introverts who reported greater imagery to concrete words rather than extroverts. The possibility of differential imagery ability in extroverts and introverts, and its role in memory, is clearly in need of much greater study. In terms of recall of meaningful material M. W. Eysenck (1976) showed that, at least with connected verbal discourse, high activation introverts produced the lowest amount of correct recalls and the greatest amount of distortion. This possibility needs to be looked at in terms of person and event memory.

A selective but representative review of relevant findings in the field of personality as indexed by introversion/extroversion, and its relationship to memory, has now been presented. The interaction is fairly well established in the area of verbal memory, it now needs to be looked at in terms of visual memory, and especially as it applies to eyewitness reliability. By extrapolation from the above studies such a dimension of individual differences would seem to be an important consideration in the understanding of person identification.

GROUP DIFFERENCES IN PERSON IDENTIFICATION – POLICE AND CIVILIANS

A recent police recruitment advertisement made the following claims: 'You will develop on the beat the ability to observe and remember. To make the seemingly unimportant stick. You will be taught to be observant and to develop a quick eye for detail.'

Is this true? Are policemen more reliable as witnesses than the ordinary man in the street? The Peter Hain case greatly stimulated interest in questions of identification, and in the Lazlo Virag case in 1969, and that of Oliver Francis (the 1976 Caribbean Club affray) policemen were among those who wrongly picked them out in identity parades. In the case of George Davis, whose appeal was disallowed, five policemen ensured the conviction of a man who failed to be identified by no less than thirty-eight other witnesses. Were the police in this case more reliable than those who proclaimed (by implication) his innocence?

The promises in the police advertisement might strengthen the layman's idea about memory and the police. The non-specialist uses the analogy of the camera or the tape recorder when he or she thinks about memory. Just as you get good or bad cameras and tapes, so (on this analogy) you get good or bad perceivers and memorizers. And traditionally the police are thought to have good powers of perception and memory. But is memory like a camera or a tape, and are the policemen better endowed with perceptual and memorial ability than the average non-policeman?

It has been argued that to remember was to have organized. But organization is not the whole story: it describes memory but does not explain it. The most recent research underlines the fact that people select what they will pay attention to and remember. It has also been found that once this selection has been made, the information is 'fixed' by embedding it in already existing knowledge structures. This means that when recall or recognition is asked for, the output is constructed from stored meanings. This process of memory can lead to error. Does it make any difference whether you are a policeman or not? It could be that police will be more prone to impute (and therefore remember) actions of a criminal nature which perhaps never even occurred, precisely because of their past training and experience.

Another potential source of error is capacity. It is generally held that man is a 'limited capacity processor'. In other words, the amount of information which he can attend to, and remember, at any one time, is quite small (hence his need to select). This can be shown in a number of ways, but chiefly by the 'span of apprehension' method. You are presented with a number of words, letters or digits and asked to repeat them back in the order given, without error. Most people can do this with six or seven items. Above seven, a large number of errors begin to appear. This psychological fact has been recognized in practical situations: it is no accident that British telephone numbers and car number plates do not exceed the magical number seven.

Very few psychological research reports on the police exist (see Clifford, 1976 for review). What does exist supports the likely validity of the two suggested sources of error outlined above.

An experiment which provides evidence that the police exhibit a limited memory capacity was one carried out by Bull and Reid (1975), designed to compare face-to-face and TV briefing sessions in terms of how much policemen and policewomen generally retained from them. In tasks similar to this ordinary men and women usually recall accurately only about seven items of information. This was precisely what Bull and Reid found with the police, also. The police retained six or seven items quite well, but with eight items, recall dropped dramatically. In terms of the basic capacity to recall units of information the police and the general public seem not to differ.

While it could be argued that the police perceive and remember events and people better it appears that they do not. Tickner and Poulton (1975) showed films of a street scene lasting for one, two or four hours, into which various events had been deliberately inserted. They showed these to twenty-four policemen and 156 civilians. The observers' task was to watch for certain people and certain kinds of action – theft, normal exchange of goods, and general anti-social behaviour. The crucial finding was that police officers reported more alleged thefts than the civilians. In true detection of people and actions, there was no difference between civilians and the police. Of additional importance was the low detection rate (31 per cent), despite the fact that photographs of the relevant 'target people' were displayed continuously under the screen. Seeing a 'softening-up' film of the relevant people before the main film only raised correct detection to 41 per cent. This applied to both the police and the other observers. It testifies to the very poor memories which all eyewitnesses actually have. Identification at night is even worse as a similar film study by Simmonds, Poulton and Tickner (1975) showed. But, of course, the most fascinating aspect of these investigations was their confirmation of the processing argument. The use of existing knowledge to select and store information brings about errors of commission, not just of omission. The policemen greatly overestimated the actual number of thefts.

The tendency of the police to recall or perceive things not actually present is found in other research. Many studies have shown that what better recall policemen have is seriously impugned by a 'confabulation factor', i.e. the filling in of gaps, or the imputation of intentions not actually present. Marshall and Hanssen (1974) have shown how the police view events in predictably different ways from non-policemen. In their study, 291 observers (including both police and civilians) were shown a forty-two-second film in which a man approached a pram, pulled down its protective net, and then walked off. As he was walking away, a woman appeared out of a house. Statements about what was observed in the film were taken both immediately and one week later. It was found that the police noted and remembered more detail, but were prone to special types of error – especially where actions were concerned. The police remembered more correct details about dress and appearance, but they recalled twice as many incorrect facts – details that were not there, events that never happened. With the actions depicted in the scene, the civilians merely reported what was there – without imputation of suspicious intent. The police, on the other hand, 'saw' more than actually happened. One in five of the policemen said that they saw the man put his hand into the pram and take the baby out! Many said they saw the woman running towards the man with a look of worry on her face. A vital supplementary finding was that while the police were better at remembering details initially (up to one minute) they made many more errors than the non-police one week later. The public remembered less initially, but forgot less over time.

This interaction between the type of observer and the time

since the incident has important implications. It obviously affects the credibility of a policeman's testimony at long delays after the initial perception. In court cases, it is assumed that it makes little difference whether it is one day, one week or one month since the police officer first witnessed the incident in question. It is held that his memory is sound over time. The evidence cited would seem to refute this empirically. Theoretically also, it is doubtful that time makes no difference, especially for policemen. One explanation of forgetting which still has value, is that it is caused by one event 'interfering' with another stored event, especially where the events are highly similar (see Chapter 2). Memory is a decision process. Man selectively attends to and stores events. The more that is stored, of a similar nature, the greater will interference be, and therefore the greater the forgetting. The policeman by the very nature of his job, is asked to selectively perceive and store many similar events for future potential usefulness, the civilian is not. Thus policemen will forget more information of a specific type, over a given length of time, than a civilian would.

There is little doubt that the time lapse between seeing the event or criminal and identifying or recalling is important, but equally important is the length of time the witness had to initially perceive the criminal. Research at the North East London Polytechnic, Psychology Department, under the first author's guidance shows this clearly. Police and civilians were asked to describe the appearance of a target whom they had been exposed to for either 15 or 30 seconds, after a 30-second delay. The length of exposure to the target was achieved by having the target either ask the time (short exposure) or ask for directions (long exposure). Only stationary police and civilians were used, and only those who really looked at the target were used in the analysis. We found that the police recalled more details of the target than did members of the public, *but* only at longer exposure durations. At short exposure durations there was absolutely no difference between the two types of observer.

So far then research suggests that police are not necessarily better than the general public at perceiving and remembering events, actions and people, except under special circumstances, and like the general public they could be prone to misinterpret events because of their past experience. 'Confabulation' is the technically correct term for the second point, but in ordinary usage it tends to mean intentional deception, so a better term is 'misinterpretation'. Memory and perception are interpretative, and the police are especially prone to such interpretative storage.

This is shown in a study by Verinis and Walker (1970), where they presented eleven scenes to a number of policemen and to an equal number of the general public, and the observers were asked to recall details of the scenes and possible intentions. There was no difference between the two groups in recalling objective detail, but the police reported significantly more 'criminal episodes'. A man walking round a corner carrying a can was interpreted by the non-police observers as having run out of petrol. The police mostly saw him as an arsonist.

Is it just junior policemen who make the mistakes? It is often thought that, with the police, the longer the service the better the powers of observation. In court there are frequent appeals to a policeman's 'length of service'. A novice policeman's testimony carries less weight than a 'twenty year man'. How valid is the deduction that longer means better? The answer seems to be: not very sound. Most of the studies cited balanced for age within police groups and found little or no evidence of better memory with increasing length of service, although Bull and Reid (1975) did find some suggestions that police in their second year of service were better recallers than those in their first year. This is not surprising to psychologists because 'experience' is a double-edged sword. The building up of stocks of knowledge, stereotypes, attitudes and values, by means of which events are perceived and stored, counterbalances any possible gain from acquiring skill, over time, in perception and memory.

In the thorny area of identifying coloured people, these points came out clearly in a study by Billig and Milner (1976). If we can loosely equate age with rank, and experience with age, then their research is evidence on the 'length of service' argument. Billig and Milner used twenty-eight policemen and policewomen drawn from the ranks of both constables and officers, who varied markedly in their experience with coloured communities in Britain. Basically, they sought to investigate whether white policemen could identify photographs of coloured people as easily as photographs of white people. For our present purposes, they found no difference between constables and officers, or between 'experienced' and 'non-experienced' police officers.

The conclusions from all these studies are clear. Despite graffiti to the contrary, policemen are first and foremost humans! They are characterized by processing and capacity limitations like any other human. Processing limitations can be overcome by both inferential and visual techniques which can be learned, but unfortunately, in the case of the police, the inferential techniques they learn are based on existing knowledge which include values, beliefs, prejudices and 'working hypotheses' about the nature of reality. However, visual scanning techniques may be less open to such distortions. It can legitimately be argued that most of the studies listed above have tested police under essentially artificial circumstances – by using photographs or videotapes. However, the whole purpose of the North East London Polytechnic study was to approximate real-life conditions by testing police on the beat and civilians in the street. The important positive finding in this study was that at sufficiently long inspection times police did out-perform the civilians. Clifford and Richards (1977) argue strongly that, providing an irreducible minimum time for viewing was not prevented, police had processing skills which could be employed and which eventuated in better recall. While it seems to be the case that techniques of visually processing people are not universally taught to police forces, it could be argued that because they are valuable, policemen develop such heuristic scanning strategies individually. The most important point to make is that when basic skills of person recognition are tested – uncontaminated by aspects of intention, prejudice and delay – those persons with learned techniques can do better than persons with no such ready-made processing strategies. It would thus seem to us mandatory that we elucidate just what are the best methods of fixating people for later recognition (and here Chapter 4 would seem highly informative), and also that employees in areas of high criminal risk, and the population in general, be made aware of, and educated in the use of, these techniques.

8 Identification parades

In 1967 the Supreme Court of the USA deemed identification parades to be a 'critical stage' in the judicial process because there was no way of 'reconstructing line-up events for the purposes of discrediting a witness's testimony at trial' (Levine and Tapp, 1973). It was suggested that the suspect in an identification parade would have a right to counsel as is the case in the United Kingdom (though here few suspects are aware of, or employ this facility). Levine and Tapp (1973) point out that, 'because of popular faith in eyewitness identification, it is probable that a positive identification often contributes to persuading the suspect (and his attorney) to plead guilty. Therefore, most often the witness is not challenged by cross-examination.'

Recently there has been much discussion concerning the value and validity of identification parades and a committee of inquiry was set up. This Devlin Committee recognized that the differences between visual and verbal processes that were discussed in Chapter 2 are relevant to criminal identification when it noted that, 'recognition depends upon the human ability to memorise a face, even when it cannot be described with any accuracy.' As Devlin put it the problem in legal settings at the moment is that, 'Evidence of recognition if accepted, proves identity, it can be attacked as false or mistaken, but if the attack fails it is enough by itself to constitute proof.' The Committee suggested that if a witness could be no surer of identification than that the suspect resembled the wanted person then such evidence is not as strong as that of recognition. This distinction has some merit but it glosses over a problem discussed in Chapter 2, namely that there is little evidence that a witness's confidence in his identification (high confidence often being taken as synonymous with correct recognition) is of any use when judging the true accuracy of the identification. We are aware that this blurring of Devlin's attempted dichotomy does nothing to aid those attempting to rationalize the legal procedures concerning identification and we are cognizant of the criticism that psychologists frequently create more problems than they solve. However, we believe that it is only by the fullest airing of psychology's findings relevant to person identification that progress can be made. Devlin noted that, 'Psychological studies of the processes of memory and recall underline the need to approach evidence of eye-witness identification with great caution', and in this chapter we shall attempt to relate available psychological knowledge to the situation of identity parades, but in so doing we will have to point out that the Devlin Committee itself has fallen foul of the belief that we can separate out 'recalling' man from 'thinking', 'feeling' and 'believing' man.

There has been much criticism recently of the practice of identification parades but we must acknowledge at the outset that a procedure whereby a witness can select from a range of persons that individual which he believes to be the criminal is essential if justice is to be done. Before the introduction of identifiction parades witnesses were often asked to pick out from those present in the court-room the person that had committed the crime. Since the suspect was frequently placed in the dock of the court this procedure had obvious limitations. However, as an illustration of how unpredictable human beings can be we have the observations of Rolph (1957) that when witnesses were asked if they could see the criminal in court they have: '(a) pointed to the Governor of Brixton Prison, (b) to a detective sergeant waiting for the clerk of the court to sign the expenses form relating to a previous case, (c) to a reporter and (d) to a probation officer'. Identification parades as presently conducted would seem to be an improvement upon the techniques of dock identification and of confrontation. However, it is possible that present procedures can be improved in the light of the information contained in this book, and the arguments to be developed below.

The first requirement for a satisfactory appraisal of identification parades is to get clear just how accurate eyewitnesses are, and how their behaviour can be assessed. In the absence of any information from actual cases we have to rely on experimental estimates, because at real identification parades the guilt or innocence of the suspect is not generally known. However, by the use of controlled experimentation the variables present in real-life situations can be partially separated out to isolate the most relevant ones and determine their effect upon accuracy. Estimates of identification vary – but the estimations are uniformly low. Buckhout, in a series of published and unpublished studies, has conducted a number of simulated crimes, and then tested eyewitness recognition in an identification parade situation. Most of these studies were discussed and detailed in Chapter 2 and for our purposes only the results will be quoted here. In 1974 Buckhout staged a classroom incident and three weeks later presented the witnesses with two videotape line-ups (one which contained the criminal and one which did not), and they were asked to pick out the criminal. Of the 54 witnesses 14 selected the correct criminal but then 7 of these 14 went on to impeach themselves by also selecting an innocent person from the 'blank' line-up. Thus only 13.5 per cent of witnesses made an error-free positive identification. It should be pointed out that the line-up comprised only five people, and there were no look-alikes – thus identification should have been very high indeed. Brown, Deffenbacher and Sturgill (1977) presented 'criminals' for twenty-five seconds inspection to a class of students and then, one week later, re-presented the witnesses with a line-up which contained these criminals. They found approximately 50 per cent correct identifications, but also an 8 per cent positive identification of a person never seen before. Thus there was a one in two chance of a criminal not being identified, and a one in twelve chance of an innocent person being accused of being a criminal. In a following experiment using less ideal viewing conditions (note that in the above experiment criminals had been viewed for twenty-five seconds!), Brown *et al.* obtained correct identifications, after eight days, of 45 per cent and more importantly, an 18 per cent false identification rate. Thus the seen criminal was likely to be identified only two and a half times more often than a person who had never been seen before. Dent and Gray (1975) ran a comparative experiment (to be discussed below) where they presented a live incident and then sought identification from line-ups or from photographs one week later. Correct identification ran at 14 per cent for line-ups and 25 per cent for photographs. The one study which shows fairly good identification accuracy under real-life viewing conditions is a study by Buckhout where the incident involved an assault on a college professor: 40 per cent correct identification was obtained, while 25 per cent of the witnesses picked out the wrong person. In this study the identification was made from photographs rather than a live line-up, but the important manipulation was 'biasing effects'. One 'biasing' manipulation was to have some of the witnesses expecting the suspect to be definitely present in the photograph spread, while the other 'biasing' condition was to have the photograph of the suspect set apart from the other photographs, either by having the photographed person wearing atypical clothes, or by having his photograph set at an angle to the rest of the photographs. These biasing manipulations accounted for a large proportion of the relatively high correct identifications.

This last study hits at the very heart of the identification parade controversy. By its very nature there are at least two sources of bias in such a situation. The first source of bias is the witness himself, while the second source resides in the selection of the other paraders, or 'distractors' (Doob and Kirshenbaum, 1973). The witness is very prone to make the assumption (justifiably) that if the police are going to all the trouble of holding a parade then they must have a suspect. Given this assumption the witness then wants to appear trustworthy and useful. Orne's (1962) research strongly suggests that witnesses will wish to 'produce good data'. This involves the witness giving a performance characteristic of an intelligent subject, and intelligence in this situation involves being consistent in the descriptions of the criminal and identifying the accused person. To aid this 'good behaviour' the witness will pick up both manifest and latent cues from the police, the suspect and other paraders. Rosenthal (1966) has clearly and repeatedly given concrete evidence that the hopes of one person can affect the behaviour of another. Over and above this 'social set', and intimately connected with it, is the fact that in the vast majority of real-life criminal episodes (and simulated crime experiments) the witness has only a partial memory of what took place and of who perpetrated the crime. This partial memory is a source of bias. Before a line-up takes place, the witness has almost certainly given a verbal description of the criminal to the police. The problem with this is that once a person makes a public commitment (official statement) that person will adhere rigidly to it (Brehm and Cohen, 1962; Kiesler, 1971), and we have already indicated the perverting effect that this can have in Chapter 6. There it was shown that witnesses will (or could) identify a person who best resembled their publicly given verbal labelling of a partially remembered face, irrespective of whether the identified person was the criminal or not.

This finding leads us into a crucially important procedural point made by Bytheway and Clark (1976). They point out that the composition of a line-up based on the Home Office recommendations of 'persons who are as far as possible the same age, height, general appearance (including standard of dress and grooming) and position in life' could be positively harmful, because it could eventuate in a line-up which would be markedly different from a line-up based on the witness's verbal description. The Home Office line-up composition stems from the suspect the police have, a better line-up composition could stem from the witnesses initial descriptions. A Home Office-police suspect generated line-up could lead to anomalies such as occurred in the Virag case where the witness was not allowed to ask the suspect to speak, despite having heard his voice, because no other participant spoke with a comparable accent, Virag being the only foreigner on the parade. A witness-generated line-up could have prevented this situation. But it goes further than this because at base a line-up is a statistical exercise whose fairness can only be judged against a metric of bias (cf. Devlin Report, 1976, p. 114, paragraph 5.31). The idea of presenting a parade is to have persons who function to distract the witness from the suspect so that the witness will not pick the suspect automatically. Thus there is some chance level at which the suspect is likely to be selected by anyone looking at the line-up. Theoretically, this chance level is $\frac{1}{n}$, where 'n' is the number of people in the line-up. This theoretical value, the probability of the accused being picked out by someone without any knowledge of the crime, works only if there is no systematic bias. Systematic bias can be detected by presenting police line-up photographs to non-involved persons and asking them, on the bases of the witnesses' verbal description, to pick out the criminal. If the subject has not seen the criminal, and there is no bias operating, then that subject should be merely guessing and should thus select the suspect at chance level only. Bob Buckhout has usefully summarized a number of studies which have scientifically assessed the presence or absence of bias in police line-ups using this method. A 24-year-old woman of Jamaican origin was robbed and raped over a period of half an hour. The victim's description was, 'Black, 5 feet 6 inches, 120 lbs, 21 years of age with a medium complexion and a moustache'. A line-up took place several months later and the suspect was identified by the victim. The line-up comprised five distractors. However, it seemed four of the distractors had darker complexions; all the distractors' clothes were different from the suspect's; and they all appeared older than the victim. When the line-up photograph was given to uninvolved college students and they were furnished with the original verbal description given by the victim and asked whom they would choose as the criminal, 72 per cent chose the suspect (chance being 16.67 per cent). This line-up, if held in Britain, would have contravened the Home Office guidelines on height (perhaps), age (perhaps), but on the other criteria it would not. The actual line-up does, however, contravene the witness's description on all counts. Another case quoted by Buckhout is that of the State of Florida vs. Richard Campbell. A sales girl gave the following description of an armed robber, 'Black, male, 5 feet 7 inches, 160 lbs, 22–24 years old, braided hair and brown eyes', and she eventually picked him out of a line-up. The scientific assessment of the degree of bias in the line-up was achieved as above by giving thirty-four students, who did not see the crime, the police line-up photograph, the witness's initial description, and asking them to pick out the criminal. On chance the suspect should have been picked only 16.67 per cent of the time. In the event he was selected by 52 per cent of the students, who heard of, but did not see, the crime. The braided hair was the chief biasing factor, which would have been matched with distractors in a line-up generated on the bases of the victim's description, but not necessarily on the bases of a line-up generated from Home Office guidelines.

Buckhout quotes a number of other such crucially important checks on line-up bias, and we have already quoted at length the study conducted by Doob and Kirshenbaum (1973), where the witness's description 'rather good-looking' clearly specified for non-witnesses (who should and could only be guessing if no bias was operating) the person to choose. The facial attractiveness crucial in this line-up just would not be considered by a Home Office based line-up. The point of all these real-life case histories is that, while admirable in themselves, the rules for generating line-up distractors must come from the witness and not from a set of guidelines which operate *in vacuo*. This is vital because the Home Office recommendations would be acceptable if their categories were the categories which witnesses use to describe seen criminals – but they are not. Different people are likely to use different categories in describing others (Dornbusch, Hastorf, Richardson, Muzzy and Vreeland, 1965). This disjunction in the labels of the Home Office and the witness can explain the odd finding that there is often little resemblance between the real criminal and the selected suspect (Wall, 1965). Scientific evidence of bias in a line-up can be easily ascertained and when it is ascertained it is found to reside partly in the way distractors are selected. Selection on the bases of witnesses' descriptions will afford police greater sensitivity and therefore certainty, although it may make their obtaining of participants more difficult. The ideal is obviously to run the two sources of construction together. Only by this approach will the innocent be freed and the guilty brought to trial. Parades are only unbiased and therefore 'fair' if the non-suspect and an innocent suspect are equally likely to be identified (wrongly) by the witness. One way of achieving this greater fairness has been outlined and elucidated above. Another possibility will now be investigated more briefly.

A suggestion that we have put forward elsewhere (Bull and Clifford, 1976) is that two parades be used, only one of which contains the suspect. As far back as 1929 the Royal Commission on Police Powers and Procedures noted that some witnesses, 'may unconsciously tend to identify the person who most resembled their recollection of the culprit disregarding, apparently, the alternative that he may not be present at all'. We have already seen how Buckhout employed two line-ups and found that half the subjects who appeared to have good memories (by positively identifying the criminal) went on to impeach themselves by selecting an innocent person from the line-up in which the criminal was not present. Thus a double parade has the dual effect of indicating unreliable witnesses and cutting down on the 'social set' or pressure on a witness to pick someone out of a parade which he (the witness) 'knows' contains a criminal suspect. Thus the main argument for a two-parade situation is that the witness is informed that in fact one of the parades may not contain a suspect. However, as Doob and Kirshenbaum (1973) suggest, that may simply be putting the pressure on the witness in a different way, because he will still assume that the suspect is in one of the line-ups. Devlin (1976, paragraph 5.57) comes to the same conclusion: they suggest that, 'pressure to pick someone out' does not exist but they go on to argue that if the suspect is not present in the first parade the witness will be 'under even more pressure to identify someone in the second parade than may now be the case with just one parade'. The question of one parade or two would seem to be in need of experimental resolution. Personal predilection, and questions of practicality should not carry the day.

A further possible refinement in the identification parade procedures is for the participants to be unaware of which of the others is the police suspect. At the present time it is frequently the case that the non-suspects know which person in the line-up is the suspect and consequently they may convey to the witness (perhaps unwittingly) this knowledge by, for example, sideglances. If the people present during the parade become more tense and attentive as the witness moves along the line towards the suspect then this would very easily be discerned by the witness. The Devlin Report makes no mention of this. To avoid this knowledge of the suspects on the part of the participants the police will have to seriously consider their methods of obtaining line-up personnel. The habit of using nearby institutions or factories not only runs the risk of all participants knowing each other but not the 'stranger in our midst', but also having distractors who are different from the suspect by virtue of being homogeneously institutionalized (e.g. dress, appearance, manner).

Such clues as to which person in the parade is the suspect coupled with the possibility that the suspect may indeed resemble the criminal but is not in fact he, are two of the reasons why the errors of recognition in identification parades are not always random. When a witness picks out one of the parade suspects it is not unusual for other witnesses to pick out the same person even though the witnesses may never have discussed the matter. The Devlin Report noted that there is a tendency, when witnesses make a mistake, for them to make the same mistake.

In the context of identification parades this finding is not all that surprising. The 1969 Home Office Circular on identification parades (which is not binding on police forces) states that, 'The suspect should be placed among persons (if practicable eight or more) who are as far as possible of the same age, height, general appearance (including standard of dress and grooming) and position of life.' This suggestion has already been criticized because it can result in bias when compared with the witness's verbal description, but here other problems will be raised in connection with it. The above suggestions concerning distractors were made largely to ensure that a witness could not pick out the suspect solely on the grounds of there being an approximate resemblance between the suspect and the criminal. Since the circular asks that an attempt be made for all the people in the line-up to look somewhat alike then the witness's task is made rather more difficult. This is one of the ways in which,

> Identification parades should be fair, and should be seen to be fair. Every precaution should be taken to see that they are so and, in particular, to exclude any suspicion of unfairness or risk of erroneous identification through the witnesses' attention being diverted specially to the suspected person instead of equally to all persons paraded.
> (Home Office Circular, 9 1969)

The problem here is that if the police's search for non-suspected people to form part of the parade has been successful in the sense that some of these persons very closely resemble the suspect, then since recognition and identification are always the result of an approximate match between the initial memory image (which fades) and subsequent perceptions of an individual, 'errors' will be very likely to occur. The police are in a difficult position here. If the non-suspects hardly resemble the suspect then the parade may be judged to have been unfairly conducted but, on the other hand, if some or all of the people in the parade look very much alike the witness will not be able to discriminate between them. It is a fact that different unrelated individuals can look very much alike. Dent and Gray (1975) provide photographs to show how close such resemblances can be and they point out that, 'whether or not the witness decides to identify someone depends not only on how closely that person resembles his memory of the criminal, but also on how close he thinks the resemblance ought to be before he makes a positive identification', and it is precisely here that the social psychological factors in an identification parade become crucial.

Brandon and Davies (1973) make the point that, 'even if the rules are strictly observed, and the parade is satisfactory in every way, all that is proved is that the person picked out looks more like the culprit than anyone else on the parade.' These authors also note that juries seem to place great faith in identification evidence but that, 'Curiously, this only works one way. Juries do not seem to place the same faith in the person who says: "This is not the man", as in the person who says: "This is the man."' Further they believe that, 'Often witnesses who fail to make an identification, or who identify the wrong man, are not called.' In its submission to the Devlin Committee the National Council for Civil Liberties (1974) made the point that it may be a drawback of the present identification parade procedure that no information is gathered concerning how sure a witness is in his identification. While (as has been pointed out in Chapter 2) there is little evidence that a witness's certainty and accuracy go hand in hand, it may be worthwhile for this suggestion to be followed up.

The extent to which the expectancies and stereotypes that were discussed in Chapter 3 can play a role in the identification parade situation has not been studied. However, with the witness being there under strong pressure to pick someone out they may have an effect. When asked to attend a parade it is likely that a witness is under the impression that a police suspect will be in the line-up. Consequently, the witness may need to be quite sure that the criminal is not present before he refuses to pick anyone out. A close resemblance may be all that the witness requires in order to make an identification and such an identification will be all the more likely to occur if the selected person has the appearance the witness expects a certain criminal to have. A person who fits the stereotype and who is not dissimilar to the witness's memory and recall of the criminal could easily be the one picked out at the parade. However, this conclusion is not in itself a criticism of identification parades since such a selection may frequently be accurate. What needs to be done with identification parades is not to dispense with them or their evidence but to reduce the margin of error to which they are prone. Such improvements can only be gained by the study of actual real-life parades. Studies employing pseudo-parades do not contain all the pressures, commitments and risks of wrongful imprisonment or of criminals going free as do their real counterparts. It would be extremely useful to courts (and to researchers) if identification parades were filmed since, as Williams and Hammelmann (1963) suggest, 'for the proper protection of the accused it is imperative that judge and jury should be placed in a position where they can properly assess and evaluate for themselves the exact positive value of evidence of identity.'

There have been some suggestions that the pressures on witnesses that exist in the parade setting might be reduced if photographs only were used. The idea is that either a batch of photographs be shown to the witness one photograph at a time, or a photograph of the whole parade be shown. Both these suggestions have some merit but they severely restrict the number of views that a witness can have of the people in the parade. In the present parade situation the witness sees the individuals from many angles and can ask them to walk or talk if required. Dent and Gray (1975) found some evidence that colour photographs of the individuals in a parade lead to a greater proportion of correct identifications than did a conventional parade. However, these authors wisely note that all participants were aware that the situation was merely an experimental one. Nevertheless, the witnesses still

> appeared embarrassed and self-conscious as they looked at the men lined up in front of them and were less willing to look at one man for a long time than were the subjects

identifying from photographs. They also appeared more anxious to end the situation quickly when faced with the men themselves, than was the case with photographs.

This could result in hasty decisions and as Garton and Allen (1972) indicate hasty decisions are less accurate. Thus, the superior performance occasioned by the photographs is more likely to be the result of the different setting in which they are viewed than it is of any other factor and this obviously has some bearing on the way that identification parades should be conducted. Levine and Tapp (1973) point out that, 'although under stress the accuracy of an identification may be reduced, the individual's need for identifying may be increased.'

Further, in the study by Dent and Gray the photographs were examined one at a time and their results may have some bearing on the suggestion that identification parades be replaced by a system in which each person who would have been a member of a traditional parade enters in turn a room where the witness is present. Thus the witness would see the people one at a time and each would leave before the next enters. The witness would not be told how many people are available for viewing and a court could note if the witness needed a second run through this sort of 'parade'. If such a system as this were adopted it would prevent non-suspects from conveying to the witness who the real suspect was and it would provide information on how readily the witness made his choice. Furthermore, since the witness would not know how many people were going to be in this 'parade' it might reduce the number of occasions upon which the witness picks out the 'best resemblance' as in a traditional parade. Also, since the 'parading' people would be seen walking this would help get over the problem of present line-ups in which the witness is asked to identify a static person, who may originally have been seen in motion, at the time of the crime.

It is our view that if society wishes to convict persons who commit crimes, and in some cases the only evidence against them is that of identification, then identification parades as presently conducted (or preferably modified in line with the suggestions which we have made) are perhaps the most efficient way of achieving this. It is worth stressing again that no type of conviction can ever be certain. As Samuel Butler said, 'Life is the art of drawing sufficient conclusions from insufficient data.' In the context of identification, society has to decide what is 'sufficient', as do the police. Identification evidence has in the past held a privileged status, which has been reduced by the Devlin Report on Evidence of Identification in Criminal Cases, and may yet require more qualification. In the past identification parade recognition has been powerful ammunition for the prosecution: perhaps now in the light of experimental findings, and real-life disclosures, it should provide nothing more than an aid to the direction of police resources in further inquiry, that is, as an aid to police investigation. The decision as to how identification parade evidence 'ought' to be used is not our province. There is, however, one question which we as psychologists must be very aware of and that is that we may be in danger of increasing the miscarriage of justice. This possibility resides in the present research being conducted into identification parades. If psychologists 'improve' the identification parade, i.e. make it less fallible, we may be in danger of creating in the minds of jurors the belief in a completely infallible identification parade. That is, the improvement in parade procedures may misguide the juror into thinking no error will or can occur. Thus a positive identification would be held to be a positive indication of guilt. The logical prior requirement is to educate the public, as we hope we have done throughout this book, that errors occur at the point of perception, during memorization and are only compounded at later, recognition, stages.

9 Conclusion: retrospect and prospect

Deese (1972) concludes his book, *Psychology as Science and Art*, by saying, 'one aspect of the future of Psychology about which we can have no doubt whatever is that its influence will grow because society has no where else to turn for guidance and direction than to the social sciences in general and psychology in particular' (p. 107). In the past half century, Deese argues, the social sciences have grown from marginal respectability in American society to positions of great power and influence. Does the same hold true of Britain?

He argues that, at least in America, society has come to depend on scientific research in psychology, and the art and judgment of psychologists in fields such as criminology. In the process of giving advice about factual matters and about ways of achieving certain goals in this area psychologists and other social scientists have been asked to commit what G. E. Moore called the naturalistic fallacy, i.e. moving from an 'is' statement to an 'ought' statement. In Britain the situation seems to be less pleasing, at least in the area of person identification.

The debate about the reliability of eyewitness testimony culminated in the publication of the Devlin Report on Evidence of Identification in Criminal Cases in 1976. While at base a sound report, it was argued (Bull and Clifford, 1976) that the most disquieting aspect of this official document was the lack of psychological evidence used to inform its recommendations. While this is disappointing from a psychologist's point of view, it is understandable – the omission merely reflected the failure of psychological research to be seen as relevant. Devlin (1976) did not neglect psychology, in fact he says, 'One of our earliest tasks was to enquire whether recent studies in forensic and general psychology threw any light on the power of recognition which would help us to determine whether in the law of evidence it should be given some special treatment' (p. 71). He concludes, however,

> it has been represented to us that a gap exists between academic research into the powers of the human mind and the practical requirements of courts of law, and the stage seems not yet to have been reached at which the conclusions of psychological research are sufficiently widely accepted or tailored to the needs of the judicial process to become the basis for procedural change.

He went on to argue that, 'the possibility should be explored of undertaking research directed to establishing ways in which the insights of psychology could be brought to bear on the conduct of identification parades and the practice of the courts in all matters relating to evidence of identification' (p. 73). Devlin here seems to be making at least six points. He seems to imply (i) that we need to distinguish between pure and applied research, (ii) that there exist 'insights' which could be profitably studied within the eyewitness arena, (iii) that research conclusions were not generally accepted, (iv) that such research as did exist was not sufficiently tailored to judicial needs, (v) that gaps exist in our knowledge in such areas, as for example, voice identification, and lastly (vi) that psychology had little to say in terms of procedural change. These six points were assessed in this book, some more fully than others, some explicitly others only implicitly. In terms of the supposed dichotomy between pure and applied research we both accepted and rejected Devlin's belief that general psychology had little to say about the applied problem of person identification. We accepted that direct extrapolation was impossible but at the same time drew heavily upon research which we believed related to, but was not directly derived from, person identification. As Warr (1973) indicates, a continuum rather than a dichotomy better describes the perspectives and operating 'domains' of different researchers. Psychologists have always been orientated to action in the sense that they have proceeded on the assumption, implicit or explicit, that their theories and empirical knowledge would eventually be applied and Maslow (1946) has argued persuasively that it is the goals or ends of psychological science which dignify and validate its methods. To operate with the belief that pure research is only concerned with considerations of formal elegance, logical rigour and inter-subject verifiability while applied research is concerned with situationally valid, socially relevant and publicly usable know-ledge is to talk only in the short term, and to talk in extremes. The distinction between pure and applied research may be a distinction without a difference – being simply a matter of degree. However, throughout the book we have stressed the need to constantly strive for more 'real-life' experimentation, and quite deliberately drew out the differences in estimates of memory capacity generated by research conducted with photo-graphs of faces and with research based upon 'simulated crime' episodes. The two estimates differ markedly and we tend to accept the lower of the two estimates, produced under 'mock crime' experimentation.

While admittedly a caricature, it can be argued that the *modus operandi* of so-called pure research is to focus on one or other aspects of a previously published report and to seek to expand, criticize and elucidate that one point. While this in and of itself was not to be deprecated it was shown to lead to a narrowing of attention, and the diverting of consideration from other possibly useful, but apparently superficially tangential, or irrelevant factors, which, if considered, could lead to other con-clusions. These neglected factors could be the insights to which Devlin referred.

A manipulated variable becomes an 'insight' when it is shown to be an important contributor of variance to the measure of interest. To this extent the definition of insight seems to be very much like the concept of reinforcement – it will always be after the fact. There are, however, a number of insights which could be argued to be trans-situational. These insights are mainly social in nature (e.g. conformity, suggestibility) and they come into opera-tion whenever individuals interact with other individuals. An-other insight which is developing a life of its own, this time from cognitive psychology, is the central role played by meaning, and the witness's prior knowledge structures, or schemata.

Conclusion: retrospect and prospect

These two basic sets of insights – one cognitive, one social – formed the foci for Chapters 2 and 3 respectively. It was argued that the well known fact of eyewitness unreliability was not simply due to inadequate lighting, malfunctioning sensory systems or the speed of events but rather that a large portion of fallibility in testimony was directly ascribable to the methods of information processing utilized by the subject. Thus selectivity was shown to be a function of past experience, and errors of commission were largely due to logical and spatial filling in, in order to render perception coherent. Memory fallibility was shown to be the rule rather than the exception because memory is a selective, decision-making process rather than a structure. To facilitate memory the witness tries to relate current input to prior knowledge, and processes the former in terms of the latter. As such we argued that irrespective of form of input the stored memory was in terms of a modality-free, abstract, conceptual representation. Further we argued that visual and verbal memory did not differ (except perhaps quantitatively) and that face memory was no different from visual memory in general. We argued that not only was memory an integral part of man's cognitive apparatus but that cognition could not be separated from feeling and believing components of the total person. To bring this into focus we then compared memory for faces presented via photographs in laboratory studies (where one sub-process can be employed independently of other sub-processes) with memory for seen 'criminals' in the more real-life setting of mock crimes (where the sub-processes are not independently operative). The latter type of study is much more relevant, and its estimates of eyewitness accuracy were not encouraging.

The social insights in Chapter 3 were highlighted by looking at the operation of stereotyping. This again testifies to the role of past experience in present perception. Here it was clearly shown that people readily ascribe traits to face photographs, and conversely readily 'conjure up' faces to fit verbal-trait descriptions. We also had occasion to see the operation of stereotypes in the situation of photo-fit construction where, being told that a photograph was of either a 'murderer' or a 'life-boat man', predisposed photo-fit constructors to construct faces to which other, non-informed, subjects then readily ascribed the very different traits or adjectives. Other social insights such as conformity, suggestibility, and non-verbal communication were documented throughout the book in such areas as testimony generation, testimony elicitation, person identification in both photograph and line-up situations, and in individual differences in witness accuracy. Thus the argument advanced throughout the book and supported by experimental evidence was that the incorporation of these insights as independent variables has produced research which is immediately seen to be relevant to judicial concerns of identification.

As can be appreciated from our conclusions so far, the Devlin Report was one of the chief stimuli for writing this book. Thus throughout we asked ourselves whether his statement that, 'the conclusions of psychological research are .. [not] .. sufficiently widely accepted or tailored to the needs of the judicial process to become the basis of procedural change' was or was not an accurate representation of the state of the art. We hope in this book that we have shown the above statement to be either not the case or at the very least a gross overstatement. Specifically, in terms of 'procedural change' we believe that Devlin's statement flies in the face of both old and modern research. Much is contained in the literature, and has been reviewed here, which implies 'ought' statements. In terms of identification it is still the case that the face is the chief means of person recognition. Research on how faces are processed, how well they are remembered, and what factors interact with these processes and capacities is well advanced. We know fairly well what features of a face are attended to; we know where emotion resides in a face, the relative weights of single features and features in combination; and the problem of understanding the gestalt properties of faces is about to be resolved. We are beginning to obtain qualitative and quantative estimates of the effect of transformations of a face between the initial perception and the eventual recognition. Very importantly in a multi-racial society we are beginning to detail the reasons why races are best at recognizing their own race faces, and poor at other-race faces, and why one other-race face is more difficult than another. Japanese faces seem somewhat problematic to both black and white subjects. If we are not solving this problem positively we are at least in a position to say what factors are not contributory.

In the troublesome area of identification parades experimental psychologists are beginning to experiment with photographs and videotapes rather than face-to-face interaction which rule out many of the difficulties people have with interactive contact. Blank line-ups (stemming from the use of 'catch trials' in Reaction Time research) hold out some promise of rendering the· identification parade fairer to the witness and the innocent suspect. Psychologists are much exercised in trying to develop alternatives to, or modifications in, this problematical area of identification parades which, unfortunately, is still one of the best identification tools we have. We devoted a fair amount of space to the thorny area of bias and pointed out that bias resides in the officers in charge of the parade, the parade distractors and the witness himself. We also tentatively suggested several possible line-up procedures which could obviate many of the above problems.

Criminal episodes, testimony elicitation and person identification rarely occur without some verbal interaction. We looked at this in two ways, first as a possible facilitating or distorting influence on memory and later identification, and second, as a possible source of later identification in voice parades. To look at the possibility of verbal influences on visual memory we reviewed the evidence that linguistic input in the form of labels and questions has been shown to be a crucial distorter or facilitator of visual memory depending on the timing, type and amount of the verbal input. In terms of voice parades we reviewed the extant literature and pointed out areas of future research and the chief questions that need attention.

Another procedural aid to police efficiency, the photo-fit, has come under the psychologist's experimental inspection. Research carried out on its efficiency has been fairly negative, in the sense that it has been shown that it does not work very well, and few, if any, psychological variables correlate with its parameters.

In the light of these findings it is difficult to see how Devlin's assertion concerning the failure of psychology to carry implications for procedural change can be substantiated. Let us now examine the last two points that Devlin makes concerning the alleged fact that 'conclusions are not generally accepted' and that 'research is not sufficiently tailored to forensic needs'. The classical, older literature (briefly reviewed in Chapter 1) was fairly consensual. The work by Whipple, Freud, Munsterberg and

Gross, together with Binet and Stern all lead to the conclusion that sense data were fallible, recall was idiosyncratic and eye-witness testimony was inherently unreliable. Thus to reach his conclusion of 'no general acceptance' Devlin could not have been looking only at classical research. It seems likely that he was juxtaposing some modern research with the old research – and here disagreements do appear. At first glance, because person identification is at-base a perceptual memory phenomenon, it would seem likely that research into pure visual memory would be useful. What does this pure visual memory research show? It indicates that visual memory is extremely good and we reviewed this evidence in Chapter 2. Allied to pure visual memory research, which used such stimulus material as pictures, drawings, and objects, another tradition has developed which again suggests very good visual memory. This tradition employs photographs of faces as stimulus material and again 'hit rates' average about 75 per cent, and further, this excellent memory persists over quite extended periods of time. Thus we have disagreement and therefore Devlin can say that findings are not generally accepted. But, and this is the point, he is juxtaposing like with unlike. The research with photographs is illegitimate evidence in the debate. Photograph research has been conducted under a paradigm which accepts a number of general and specific simplifying assumptions. These simplifying assumptions operate at the meta-theoretical, theoretical and practical level. Thus photograph research tacitly assumes that language, memory and perception are separate and separable, that one can dissociate thinking, feeling and believing man. At the lower levels, simplifying procedures have created unreality by overly long exposure times, non-aroused subjects, and isomorphic relationships between situations of viewing and situations of recognizing or recalling.

Thus the psychological research which looks at visual memory *could* be (wrongly) said to lack coherence, but the argument is even more subtle than that because while Devlin is using modern research to deny acceptance of conclusions, he also argues that this modern research is not sufficiently tailored to the needs of the judicial process. However, Devlin has been poorly counselled – hence our original (Bull and Clifford, 1976) criticism of the report as being psychologically light – because there is another line of research which is both old and new, which is consensual and tailored. Devlin all but ignores this line. This other research tradition is the 'event', 'mock crime' or 'simulated crime' paradigm. As we pointed out the 'event' experiment was devised by Stern (1903), picked up by Kobler (1915) and Marston (1924), and developed by Buckhout (e.g. 1974) and Loftus (e.g. 1975) in America and is being developed in England at the North East London Polytechnic, and to a lesser extent, at Nottingham University by Helen Dent. The 'event' experiment has always indicated that eyewitness memory is poor, but it has very positive aspects as well. It more or less approximates real-life situations, it can easily allow the manipulation of the insights Devlin talked about and, most importantly, it allows investigations of variables which would be impossible with photographs. Thus a paradigm does exist which could serve as a bridge between the psychologist and the law enforcement agencies and it is with the simulated crime methodology that we believe the future applicability of psychology to person identification lies.

THE FUTURE

The findings outlined and discussed in this book amount to a large plus for psychology, but much remains to be done at all levels. Guidelines in the choice of problems are needed to help not only researchers, but also teachers of research, thesis supervisors, funding agencies and all concerned with research in this area. In all cases Webb (1961) suggests that three criteria must be employed in guiding research in whatever area – knowledge, dissatisfaction and generalizability. These are admirable starting points and eventual goals but the first step in an actual research undertaking is to delineate the problem to be investigated. This step is an obvious one but the actual process of decision is often difficult – the realms of possibility for research seem overwhelming. Possible research areas have been rendered manageable by Buckhout (1974) who has argued that the following three main areas of identification evidence require further clarification: (1) the initial situation, (2) the individual perceiver and memorizer, and (3) the eventual situation of recollection. There are other ways of developing a research programme such as a focus on situational, social and personality factors in eyewitness reliability but such decisions are individual affairs, guided by Webb's criteria. What is more exciting is that a number of research centres in Britain have made their choice and are already conducting or are about to launch research which cannot fail to provide useful evidence on person identification. Aberdeen University, having extensively researched the photo-fit technique, are now seeking new ways of identifying just what it is that people do when they encode a face and try to recall it. A large growth area here is obviously that of multi-dimensional scaling. Newcastle University likewise is attempting to develop a new tool for use by police which could possibly supplant the use of photo-fit. Nottingham University is taking a new tack and looking at children's testimony under a variety of situations of viewing, interrogation and recall. Cambridge University is busily working on the real problem of why, and what happens when, recognition fails. The North East London Polytechnic is currently engaged in a research programme which hopes to elucidate the effect of certain social, situational and personality factors in eyewitness testimony.

The number of undergraduate students from various departments who are conducting projects in identification problems, and the increase in the frequency of research seminars being held at universities, all serve to indicate a ground swell. The entry of the SSRC and the Home Office as grant awarding bodies simply underlines this.

Thus the Devlin Report may have been over pessimistic i.. its conclusions concerning the extent and validity of psychology's contribution, but when we look to the future there are a number of crucial points which still need intensive debate before we can conclude that all is well. These problems involve the possibility of educating the public in matters of person identification, the possibility of psychological findings sometimes being of disservice to law enforcement (as discussed in Chapter 8), and lastly, the need on the part of psychologists to undertake a reorientation in their experimentation. One of the latent functions of this book has been to educate the 'man in the street', that is, the potential victim, eyewitness or juror, and thus help develop what Bermant, Nemeth and Vidmar (1976) refer to as external legal socialization. These authors define external legal socialization as 'the development of legal attitudes and behaviour within the general population'. We hope we have done this in terms of potential victims by outlining the best methods of processing a face, by outlining ways in which distorted testimony can be prevented on the part of an eyewitness, and by suggesting that jurors ought in certain cases to be much more sceptical of the validity of eyewitness testimony. Specifically, throughout the book we indicated how specific features and features in combination differentially contribute to identification accuracy, how faces are best scanned for better fixation in memory, and how an adequate label can help, but also how an inadequate label can hinder, accuracy. We have strongly hinted that victims and bystanders should try to be cognizant of prejudices and stereotypes and that different-race faces may require different processing than own-race faces for best memory.

In terms of jurors we have provided information on how difficult it is for a person to really remember another person, or a series of actions or verbal statements which occurred during a criminal episode. We indicated, and elaborated upon, the fact that person identification, which intuitively seems so easy is in fact a very difficult process because by their very nature perception and memory are error-prone mechanisms, and thus inaccuracy can enter at any and all of three stages (the situation of viewing, the memorization phase, or the situation of identification). The only safe conclusion is that the weight of evidence strongly suggests that in real-life situations eyewitness testimony and identification are not infallible. This must be realized by jurors. Gone are the days when man could comfortably be viewed as a tape recorder or a videotape. Gone also is the gullibility of jurors in the face of such statements as 'I will never forget his face' or the credulity of perfect perception of a person's face in the light cast by a gun's discharge. We have summarized the research which shows that the higher the emotional loading of an incident the poorer the perception and memory of it (and not vice versa as was commonly believed). We also quoted studies which indicate no relationship, or in fact an inverse relationship, between confidence of correctness and objectively verifiable correctness.

As we have stated, the juror is, in the last analysis, the judge of fact. What we have tried to assert is that 'fact' is not black or white, either-or, rather it is a very extended continuum of grey. Fallibility resides in (a) the witness for cognitive and social reasons, (b) in the situation of viewing, (c) in the situation of recollection, and (d) in the situation of identification. Perception in criminal episodes is a 'one shot' phenomenon, but person identification is not. It is multifaceted and multidetermined. Our brief was to lay bare certain of these facets and factors. By so doing we hope we have sown seeds both of doubt and of hope: doubt that eyewitness identification can hereafter be held to be a 'simple affair'; hope in that perhaps by knowledge of the causes of faulty perception and memory, located as they are in cognitive and social domains, victims will be better prepared to process information about his or her attacker, eyewitnesses will be better prepared against distortion by self and by others, and that jurors will be better able to judge credibility because they will have some insight into what person identification really involves.

There is, however, a nagging doubt which we personally do not hold, but which we know others do. This doubt is that by a serious intention to facilitate the prosecution of the guilty and the exoneration of the innocent we may in fact be creating more problems than we are solving: that we may actually be increasing the potential for miscarriage of justice. It could be argued that we have suggested very few principles for practice, that is, that we have not been concerned with policy research (Wilson, 1975). This claim is completely justifiable and was a deliberate intention on our part. As scientists we are concerned with questions of 'is', not of 'ought'. Thus our book has been a sustained causal analysis rather than a policy analysis of person identification. We have been concerned to look at the causes of faulty person recognition rather than provide psychologically based policy recommendations for both police and law officials. And yet by looking at 'is' questions one almost inescapably becomes concerned with 'ought' statements. This is most clearly seen in Chapter 8 where policy statements almost appeared explicitly. Implicit policy recommendations appear in every chapter, and are there for any psycho-legal reader to pick up. However, our main aim was to point out and point up the desirability of maximizing verisimilitude in the experimental setting, and to stress caution in generalizing from laboratory based, non-emotional situations to real-life, emotion laden, fast-moving and often brief eyewitness occasions. A prerequisite of policy recommendations is the development of a body of research data and hypotheses based on policy-relevant legal issues. We have, at various places throughout the book, indicated where further research is necessary and ought to proceed with all haste. In the absence of this data bank, policy statements are open to the attack of superficiality, impracticality, and woolly-headed theoretical nonsense. We believe that the growth in psycho-legal reciprocity will occur only if psychologists are willing to take a long hard look at just what they are doing and not doing, both in the long and the short term. We have been very concerned to stress that psychology, as it exists at the moment, has a great deal to offer in the way of clarification and understanding of person identification. It could do much more. As Littman (1961) laconically stated, when other professions come to psychology for help 'they are disappointed and indeed often aggrieved. What they begin to read with enthusiasm, they put down with depression. What seems promising turns out to be sterile, trivial or false, and, in any case, a waste of time'. Now this may be as much an indictment of the 'other professions' as of psychology but it is also, we think, a comment on the orientation of much of our psychological experimentation. The question we must ask ourselves is whether our orientation is in need of alteration. As we have argued, pure researchers are necessary, but they are not sufficient. Applied research of a *really* applied nature is badly needed. Future research must build upon all that has gone before but must now shift the focus a little, and at least ask itself, 'would these (pure) results be produced in a more "open" (applied) situation?' Future basic research is needed into the factors that influence individual identification but the challenge to experimental and social psychology is clear. Boring (1950) pointed out that although Hugo Munsterberg applied the psychology of his day to courtroom practices as early as 1907, the idea and the lead did not catch on, and in fact his effort brought him only disfavour from the rest of the psychological establishment. We have attempted to bring the theoretical and practical knowledge of present day psychology, seventy years later, to bear on a more circumscribed area of psycho-legal concern but we hope that this time the lead is taken up. We appreciate that our psychological policies may be unpalatable to a large number of psychologists but in this psycho-legal area, perhaps more than in any other, we already possess the theory and method to make important practical contributions. If we have gone some way to generate interest, kindle enthusiasm and sharpen resolve in this area we will have achieved at least part of what we set out to do.

Bibliography

ABERNETHY, E. (1940), 'The effect of changed environmental conditions upon the results of college examinations,' *Journal of Psychology, 10*, 293–301.

ADCOCK, C. and WEBBERLEY, M. (1971), 'Primary mental abilities', *Journal of General Psychology, 84*, 229–43.

AIKEN, L. (1963), 'The relationships of dress to selected measures of personality in undergraduate women', *Journal of Social Psychology, 59*, 119–28.

ALEXANDER, N., cited in A. Goldstein (in press), *Eyewitness identification: A psychologist's View.*

ALLEN, A. (1950), *Personal Descriptions*, Butterworth, London.

ALLPORT, G. (1924), 'Eidetic imagery', *British Journal of Psychology, 15*, 99–120.

ALLPORT, G. (1928), 'The eidetic image and the after image', *American Journal of Psychology, 40*, 418–25.

ALLPORT, G. (1937), *Personality: A Psychological Interpretation*, Constable, London.

ALLPORT, G. and VERNON, P. (1933), *Studies in Expressive Movements*, Macmillan, London.

ALPER, A., BUCKHOUT, R., CHERN, S., HARWOOD, R. and SLOMOVITS, M. (1976), 'Eyewitness identification: accuracy of individual vs. composite recollection of a crime', *Bulletin of the Psychonomic Society, 8*, 147–9.

ANDERSON, J. and BOWER, G. (1972), 'Recognition and retrieval processes in free recall', *Psychological Review, 79*, 97–123.

ANDERSON, N. (1965), 'Primacy effects in personality impression formation using a generalized order effect paradigm', *Journal of Personality and Social Psychology, 2*, 1–9.

ANNETT, M. (1970), 'The growth of manual preference and speed', *British Journal of Psychology, 61*, 545–58.

ARGYLE, M. (1969), *Social Interaction*, Tavistock Publications, London.

ARNHEIM, R. (1949), 'The Gestalt theory of expression', *Psychological Review*, *56*, 156–71.

ATKINSON, J. and WALKER, E. (1955), 'The affiliation motive and perceptual sensitivity to faces', *Journal of Abnormal and Social Psychology*, *53*, 38–41.

BADDELEY, A. (1976), *The Psychology of Memory*, Harper, New York.

BAGGETT, P. (1975), 'Memory for implicit and explicit information in pictures', *Journal of Verbal Learning and Verbal Behaviour*, *14*, 538–48.

BAHRICK, H., BAHRICK, P. and WITTLINGER, R. (1975), 'Fifty years of memory for names and faces: a cross-sectional approach', *Journal of Experimental Psychology: General*, *104*, 54–75.

BAHRICK, H. and BOUCHER, B. (1968), 'Retention of visual and verbal codes of the same stimuli', *Journal of Experimental Psychology*, *78*, 417–22.

BAILEY, W., SHINEDLING, M. and PAYNE, R. (1970), 'Obese individuals' perception of body image', *Perceptual and Motor Skills*, *31*, 617–18.

BAKER, E. (1967), 'Perceiver variables involved in the recognition of faces', unpublished doctoral dissertation, University of London.

BARON, J. and THURSTON, I. (1973), 'An analysis of the word-superiority effect', *Cognitive Psychology*, *4*, 207–28.

BARTHOLOMEUS, B. (1973), 'Voice identification by nursery school children', *Canadian Journal of Psychology*, *27*, 464–72.

BARTLETT, F. (1932), *Remembering: a Study in Experimental and Social Psychology*, Cambridge University Press.

BAY, E. (1953). 'Disturbances of visual perception and their examination', *Brain*, *76*, 515–50.

BEGG, I. (1971), 'Recognition memory for sentence meaning and wording', *Journal of Verbal Learning and Verbal Behaviour*, *10*, 114–19.

BEIER, E. (1952), 'The effect of induced anxiety on flexibility of intellectual functioning', *Psychological Monographs*, 326.

BEIJK-DOCTER, M. and ELSHOUT, J. (1969), 'Valdafhan kelij kheid en geheugen met betrekking tot sociaal relevant en sociaal niet-relevant materiaal', *Nederlands Tijdschrift voor de Psychologie enhaar Grensgebieden*, *24*, 267–79.

BELBIN, E. (1950), 'The influence of interpolated recall upon recognition', *Quarterly Journal of Experimental Psychology*, *2*, 163–9.

BELBIN, E. (1956), 'The effect of propaganda on recall, recognition and behaviour', *British Journal of Psychology*, *47*, 163–74.

BERELSON, B. and SALTER, P. (1946), 'Majority and minority Americans', *Public Opinion Quarterley*, *10*, 168–90.

BERGER, D. (1969), 'They all look alike to me', unpublished doctoral dissertation, Vanderbilt University, Tennessee.

BERMANT, G., NEMETH, C. and VIDMAR, N. (1976), *Psychology and the Law*, Lexington Books, Toronto.

BERRIEN, F. (1955), 'Psychology and the Court', in G. Dudycha (ed.), *Psychology for Law Enforcement Officials*, C. C. Thomas, Springfield, Illinois.

BEVAN, W., SECORD, P. and RICHARDS, J. (1956), 'Personalities in faces: (v) Personal identification and the judgement of facial characteristics', *Journal of Social Psychology, 44,* 289–91.

BIEDERMAN, I. (1972), 'Perceiving real-world scenes', *Science, 177,* 77–80.

BIEDERMAN, I., GLASS, A. and STACY, E. (1973), 'Searching for objects in real-world scenes', *Journal of Experimental Psychology, 97,* 22–7.

BILLIG, M. and MILNER, D. (1976), 'A spade is a spade in the eyes of the law', *Psychology Today, 2,* 13–15, 62.

BINET, A. (1897),'Description d'un objet', *L'Année Psychologique, 3,* 296.

BINET, A. (1900), *La Suggestibilité,* Schleicher Frères, Paris.

BIRDWHISTELL, A. (1971), *Kinesics and Context,* Allen Lane the Penguin Press, London.

BLAKEMORE, C. (1973), 'Environmental constraints on development in the visual system', in R. Hinde and J. Stevenson-Hinde, (eds), *Constraints on Learning,* Academic Press, London and New York.

BLOCK, E. (1975), *Voiceprinting,* McKay, New York.

BOBROW, G. and BOWER, G. (1969), 'Comprehension and recall of sentences', *Journal of Experimental Psychology, 80,* 455–61.

BOLT, R., COOPER, F., DAVID, E., DENES, P., PICKETT, J. and STEVENS, K. (1969), 'Speaker identification by speech spectrograms: a scientist's view of its reliability for legal purposes', *Journal of the Accoustical Society of America, 47,* 597–612.

BOND, E. (1972), 'Perception of form by the human infant', *Psychological Bulletin, 77,* 225–45.

BORG, G., EDGREN, B. and MARKLAND, G. (1973), 'The reliability and stability of the indicators in a simple walk test', *Reports from the Institute of Applied Psychology, University of Stockholm,* no. 35.

BORING, E. (1950), *A History of Experimental Psychology,* Appleton-Century-Crofts, New York.

BORTZ, J. (1970), 'On the reciprocal relationships between rating of speakers voices and the voice of the rater', *Archiv für Psychologie, 122,* 231–48.

BOURNE, L. (1966), *Human Conceptual Behaviour,* Allyn & Bacon, New York.

BOWER, G. (1972), 'Mental imagery and associative learning', in L. Gregg (ed.), *Cognition and Learning,* Wiley, New York.

BOWER, G. and KARLIN, M. (1974), 'Depth of processing pictures of faces and recognition memory', *Journal of Experimental Psychology, 103,* 751–7.

BRADSHAW, J. (1969), 'The information conveyed by varying the dimensions of features in human outline faces', *Perception and Psychophysics, 6,* 5–9.

BRADSHAW, J. and MCKENZIE, B. (1971), 'Judging outline faces: a developmental study', *Child Development, 42,* 929–37.

BRADSHAW, J. and WALLACE, G. (1971), 'Models for the processing and identification of faces', *Perception and Psychophysics, 9,* 443–7.

BRANDON, R. and DAVIES, C. (1973), *Wrongful Imprisonment,* Allen & Unwin, London.

BREHM, J. and COHEN, A. (1962), *Explorations in Cognitive Dissonance*, Wiley, New York.

BRICKER, P. and PRUZANSKY, S. (1966), 'Effects of stimulus content and duration on talker identification', *Journal of the Accoustical Society of America, 40,* 1441–9.

BRITISH ASSOCIATION FOR THE ADVANCEMENT OF SCIENCE (1974), *Science and the Police.*

BROADBENT, D. (1971), *Decision and Stress*, Academic Press, London and New York.

BROOKS, R. and GOLDSTEIN, A. (1963), 'Recognition by children of inverted faces', *Child Development, 34,* 1033–44.

BROWN, E., DEFFENBACHER, K. and STURGILL, W. (1977), 'Memory for faces and the circumstances of encounter', *Journal of Applied Psychology.*

BROWN, R. (1958), *Words and Things*, Illinois Press, Glencoe.

BROWN, R. (1965), *Social Psychology*, Free Press, New York.

BROWN, R. and MCNEILL, D. (1964), 'The "tip of the tongue" phenomena', *Journal of Verbal Learning and Verbal Behaviour, 5,* 325–37.

BRUCHON, M. (1969), 'L'amplitudegestuelle et la personalité' (gestural amplitude and personality), *Bulletin de Psychologie, 23,* 426–7.

BRUNER, J. (1958), 'Social psychology and perception', in E. Maccoby, T. Newcombe and E. Hartley (eds), *Readings in Social Psychology*, Henry Holt, New York.

BRUNER, J., (1961), 'The act of discovery', *Harvard Educational Review, 31,* 21–32.

BRUNER, J. (1974), *Beyond the Information Given: Studies in the Psychology of knowing*, Allen & Unwin, London.

BRUNER, J., BUSIEK, R. and MINTURN, A. (1952), 'Assimilation in the immediate reproduction of visually perceived figures', *Journal of Experimental Psychology, 44,* 151–5.

BRUNER, J. GOODNOW, J. and AUSTIN, G. (1956), *A Study of Thinking*, Wiley, New York.

BRUNER, J. and POSTMAN, L. (1949), 'On the perception of incongruity: a paradigm', *Journal of Personality, 18,* 206–23.

BRUNER, J., SHAPIRO, D. and TAGIURI, R. (1958), 'The meaning of traits in isolation and in combination', Chapter 18 of R. Tagiuri and L. Petrullo (eds), *Person Perception and Interpersonal Behaviour*, Stanford University Press.

BRUNSWIK, E. (1956), *Perception and the Representative Design of Psychological Experiments*, University of California Press.

BUCKHOUT, R. (1974a), 'Determinants of eyewitness performance in a line-up', Report no. CR-9, *Center for Responsive Psychology*, New York.

BUCKHOUT, R. (1974b), 'Eyewitness testimony', *Scientific American, 231,* 23–31.

BUCKHOUT, R. (1975a), 'Nearly 2000 witnesses can be wrong', Report no. CR-22 July, *Center for Responsive Psychology*, New York.

Bibliography

BUCKHOUT, R. (1975b), 'The psychology of eyewitness testimony', *Law and Psychology Review*, *1*, 75–91.

BUCKHOUT, R. and FIGUEROA, D. (1974), 'Eyewitness identification', Report no. CR-11, *Center for Responsive Psychology*, New York.

BULL, R. (1974), 'The importance of being beautiful', *New Society*, *30*, 412–14.

BULL, R. (1975), 'Psychology, fashion and clothing: a review', *Bulletin of the British Psychological Society*, *28*, 459–65.

BULL, R. and CLIFFORD, B. (1976), 'Identification: the Devlin Report', *New Scientist*, *70*, 307–8.

BULL, R. and REID, R. (1975), 'Recall after briefing: television versus face-to-face presentation', *Journal of Occupational Psychology*, *48*, 73–8.

BULL, R. and STEVENS, J. (in press), 'The effects of attractiveness of writer and penmanship on essay grades'.

BURTT, M. (1931), *Legal Psychology*. Prentice-Hall, Englewood Cliffs.

BUTCHER, H. (1968), *Human Intelligence*, Methuen, London.

BYTHEWAY, W. and CLARK, M. (1976), 'The conduct and uses of identification parades', *Journal of Criminal Law*, July.

CADY, H. (1924), 'On the psychology of testimony', *American Journal of Psychology*, *35*, 110-12.

CARMICHAEL, L., HOGAN, H. and WALTER, A. (1932), 'An experimental study of the effect of language on the reproduction of visually perceived form', *Journal of Experimental Psychology*, *15*, 73–86.

CARMICHAEL, L., ROBERTS, S. and WESSELL, N. (1937), 'A study of the judgement of manual expression as presented in still and motion pictures', *Journal of Social Psychology*, *8*, 115–42.

CARON, A., CARON, R., CALDWELL, R. and WEISS, S. (1973), 'Infant perception of the structural properties of the face', *Developmental Psychology*, *9*, 385–99.

CARPENTER, G. (1974), 'Mothers' faces and the newborn', *New Scientist*, *61*, 809, 742–4.

CARPENTER, G., TECCE, J., STECHLER, G. and FRIEDMAN, S. (1970), 'Differential visual behaviour to human and humanoid faces in early infancy', *Merrill-Palmer Quarterly*, *16*, 91–108.

CARROLL, J. (1964), *Language and Thought*, Prentice-Hall, Englewood Cliffs.

CAVIOR, H., HAYES, S. and CAVIOR, N. (1975), 'Physical attractiveness of female offenders', in A. Brodsky (ed.), *The Female Offender*, Sage Publications, London.

CHANCE, J. and GOLDSTEIN, A. (1976), 'Recognition of faces and verbal labels', *Bulletin of Psychonomic Society*, *7*, 384–7.

CHANCE, J., GOLDSTEIN, A. and MCBRIDE, L. (1975), 'Differential experience and recognition memory for faces', *Journal of Social Psychology*, *97*, 243–53.

CHANCE, J., GOLDSTEIN, A. and SCHICHT, W. (1967), 'Effects of acquaintance and friendship on children's recognition of classmates' faces', *Psychonomic Science*, *7*, 223–4.

222

CHAPMAN, R. (1975), 'A pilot study of a method for testing the public image of forms of transport', *Working paper no. 10 of Transport Operations Research Group*, University of Newcastle.

CHILD, I. (1936), 'The judging of occupations from printed photographs', *Journal of Social Psychology*, 7, 117–18.

CHOMSKY, N. (1957), *Syntactic Structures*, Mouton, The Hague.

CHOMSKY, N. (1965), *Aspects of the Theory of Syntax*, M.I.T. Press, Cambridge, Mass.

CLARK, H. and CHASE, W. (1972), 'On the process of comparing sentences against pictures', *Cognitive Psychology*, 3, 472–517.

CLEETON, G. and KNIGHT, F. (1924), 'Validity of character judgements based on external criteria', *Journal of Applied Psychology*, 8. 215–31.

CLIFFORD, B. (1975), 'The case of mistaken identities', *Psychology Today*, 1, 15–19, 58.

CLIFFORD, B. (1976), 'The police as eyewitnesses', *New Society*, 36, 707, 176–7.

CLIFFORD, B. and COLLIER, A. (in preparation), 'A continuum of certainty vs. a dual encoding hypothesis'.

CLIFFORD, B. and HOLLIN, C. (in press), 'Individual and situational factors in eyewitness testimony', *Journal of Applied Psychology*, 1978, 63.

CLIFFORD, B. and RICHARDS, G. (1977), Comparison of recall by police and civilians under conditions of long and short durations of exposure', *Perceptual and Motor Skills*, 45, 503–12.

CLIFFORD, B. and SCOTT, J. (in preparation), 'The effect of nature of crime on male and female eyewitnesses' recall of actions, descriptions and verbal information.'

CLIFFORD, M. and WALSTER, E. (1973), 'The effect of physical attractiveness on teacher expectation', *Sociology of Education*, 46, 248–58.

COHEN, R. (1966), 'Effect of verbal labels on the recall of a visually perceived simple figure: recognition vs. reproduction', *Perceptual and Motor Skills*, 23, 859–62.

COHEN, R. (1967), 'Interaction between a visually perceived simple figure and an appropriate verbal label in recall', *Perceptual and Motor Skills*, 24, 287–92.

COHEN, R. (1973), *Patterns of Personality Judgement*, Academic Press, New York and London.

COHEN, R. and GRANSTROM, K. (1970), 'Reproduction and recognition in short-term visual memory', *Quarterly Journal of Experimental Psychology*, 22, 450–7.

COLE, P. and PRINGLE, P. (1974), *Can You Positively Identify This Man? George Ince and the Barn Murder*, Deutsch, London.

COLTHEART, M. (1975), 'Faces', *New Behaviour*, 2, 14–15.

COMPTON, N. (1962), 'Personal attributes of colour and design preferences in clothing fabrics', *Journal of Psychology*, 54, 191–5.

CRAIK, F. and LOCKHART, R. (1972), 'Levels of processing: a framework for memory research', *Journal of Verbal Learning and Verbal Behaviour*, 11, 671–84.

Bibliography

CROSS, J., CROSS, J. and DALY, J. (1971), 'Sex, race, age and beauty as factors in recognition of faces', *Perception and Psychophsics, 10,* 393–6.

CROWNE, D. and MARLOW, D. (1964), *The Approval Motive,* Wiley, New York.

CRUTCHFIELD, R., WOODWORTH, D. and ALBRECHT, R. (1958), 'Perceptual performance and the effective person', USAF WADC, *Technical Note,* nos. 58–60.

CUTLER, P., THIGPEN, C., YOUNG, T. and MUELLER, E. (1972), 'The evidentiary value of spectrographic voice identification'. *Journal of Criminal Law, Criminology and Police Science, 63,* 343–55.

DANIEL, T. and ELLIS, H. C. (1972), 'Stimulus codability and long term recognition memory for visual form', *Journal of Experimental Psychology, 93,* 83–9.

DANNENMAIER, W. and THUMIN, F. (1964), 'Authority status as a factor in perceptual distortion of size', *Journal of Social Psychology, 63,* 361–5.

DARNBROUGH, M. A. (1977), 'A Survey on the Use of Photo-fit in England and Wales', Home Office, © Crown Copyright.

DAVIES, G. (1969), 'Recognition memory for pictured and named objects', *Journal of Experimental Child Psychology, 7,* 448–58.

DAVIES, G., MILNE, J. and GLENNIE, B. (1973), 'On the significance of 'double encoding' for the superior recall of pictures to names', *Quarterley Journal of Experimental Psychology, 25,* 413–33.

DEBUS, R. (1970), 'Effects of brief observation of model behaviour on Conceptual tempo of impulsive children', *Developmental Psychology, 2,* 22–32.

DEESE, J. (1972), *Psychology as Science and Art,* Harcourt Brace Jovanovich, New York.

DENES, P. (1974), 'Speech recognition: old and new ideas', in D. Reddy (ed.), *Speech Recognition,* Academic Press, New York and London.

DENT, H. and GRAY, F. (1975), 'Identification on parade', *New Behaviour, 1,* 366–9.

DE RENZI, E. and SPINNLER, H. (1966), 'Facial recognition in brain damaged patients', *Neurology, 16,* 145–52.

DE VARIS, D. (unpublished), cited in S. Messick and F. Damarin, 'Cognitive style and memory for faces', *Journal of Abnormal and Social Psychology, 69,* 313–18.

DEVLIN REPORT (1976), *Report to the Secretary of State for the Home Department of the Departmental Committee on Evidence of Identification in Criminal Cases,* HMSO, London.

DILLON, D. (1962), 'Measurement of perceived body size', *Perceptual and Motor Skills, 14,* 191–6.

DION, K. (1972), 'Physical attractiveness of children's transgressions', *Journal of Personality and Social Psychology, 24,* 207–13.

DOOB, A. and KIRSHENBAUM, H. (1973), 'Bias in police line-ups – partial remembering', *Journal of Police Science and Administration, 1,* 287–93.

DORNBUSCH, S., HASTORF, A., RICHARDSON, S., MUZZY, R. and
VREELAND, R. (1965), 'The perceiver and the perceived: their relative
influence on the categories of interpersonal cognition', *Journal of
Personality and Social Psychology, 1*, 434–40.

DUCHARME, R. and FRAISSE, P. (1965), 'Etude genétique de la
mémorisation de mots et d'images', *Canadian Journal of Psychology,
19*, 253–61.

DUNAWAY, D. (1973), An unpublished research paper cited in E. Green,
Psychology for Law Enforcement, Wiley, New York, 1976.

EBBINGHAUS, H. (1885), *Über das Gedächtnis*, Dunker, Leipzig:
H. Ruyer and C. E. Bussenius (translation), *Memory*, Teachers
College Press, New York, 1913.

EDWARDS, A. (1941), 'Political frames of reference as a factor
influencing recognition', *Journal of Abnormal Psychology, 36*,
35–40.

EDWARDS, J. (1973), 'The status of voiceprints as admissible evidence',
Syracuse Law Review, 24, 1261–78.

EFRAN, L. (1974), 'The effect of physical appearance on the judgement
of guilt, interpersonal attraction, and severity of recommended
punishment in a simulated jury task', *Journal of Research in
Personality, 8*, 45–54.

EISENBERG, P. (1937), 'A further study in expressive movement',
Character and Personality, 5, 296–301.

EISENBERG, P. and REICHLINE, P. (1939), 'Judging expressive
movement: II. Judgements of dominance-feeling from motion
pictures of gait', *Journal of Social Psychology, 10*, 345–57.

EKMAN, P. and FRIESEN, W. (1969), 'Non-verbal leakage and clues to
deception', *Psychiatry, 32*, 88–106.

EKMAN, P., FRIESEN, W. and ELLSWORTH, P. (1972), *Emotion in the
Human Face*, Pergamon Press, New York.

ELLIOT, R. and MCMICHAEL, R. (1963), 'Effects of specific training on
form dependence', *Perceptual and Motor Skills, 17*, 363–7.

ELLIOTT, E., WILLS, E. and GOLDSTEIN, A. (1973), 'The effect of
discrimination training on the recognition of white and oriental
faces', *Bulletin of Psychonomic Society, 2*, 71–3.

ELLIS, H. C. (1968), 'Transfer of stimulus predifferentiation to shape
recognition and identification learning: the role of properties of
verbal labels', *Journal of Experimental Psychology, 78*, 401–9.

ELLIS, H. C. (1972), 'Verbal processes in the encoding of visual pattern
information: an approach to language, perception and memory', in
M. Meyer (ed.), *Third Western Symposium on Learning: Cognitive
Learning*, Western Washington State College, Bellingham.

ELLIS, H. D. (1975), 'Recognizing faces', *British Journal of Psychology,
66*, 409–26.

ELLIS, H. D., DEREGOWSKI, J. and SHEPHERD, J. (1975), 'Descriptions
of white and black faces by white and black subjects', *International
Journal of Psychology, 10*, 119–23.

Bibliography

ELLIS, H. D., SHEPHERD, J. and BRUCE, A. (1973), 'The effect of age and sex upon adolescents' recognition of faces', *Journal of Genetic Psychology*, *123*, 173–4.

ELLIS, H. D., SHEPHERD, J. and DAVIES, G. (1975), 'An investigation of the use of the photo-fit technique for recalling faces', *British Journal of Psychology*, *66*, 29–37.

EXLINE, R. (1963), 'Exploration in the process of person perception: visual interaction in relation to competition sex and need for approval', *Journal of Personality*, *31*, 1–20.

EYSENCK, H. (1947), *Dimensions of Personality*, Routledge & Kegan Paul, London.

EYSENCK, H. (1953), *The Structure of Human Personality*, Methuen, London.

EYSENCK, M. W. (1976), 'Extroversion, verbal learning and memory', *Psychological Bulletin*, *83*, 75–90.

FAGAN, J. (1972), 'Infants' recognition memory for faces', *Journal of Experimental Child Psychology*, *14*, 453–76.

FAGAN, J. (1973), 'Infants' delayed recognition memory and forgetting', *Journal of Experimental Child Psychology*, *16*, 424–50.

FAGAN, J. (1976), 'Infants' recognition of invariant features of faces', *Child Development*, *47*, 627–38.

FANTZ, R. (1961), 'The origins of form perception', *Scientific American*, *204*, 66–72.

FANTZ, R., FAGAN, J. and MIRANDA, S. (1975), 'Early perceptual development as shown by visual discrimination, selectivity and memory with varying stimulus and population parameters', in L. Cohen and P. Salapatek (eds), *Infant Perception: from Sensation to Cognition: Basic Visual Processes*, vol. 1, Academic Press, New York and London.

FAST, J. (1971), *Body Language*, Souvenir Press, London.

FAUST, C. (1947), cited in H. Ellis, 'Recognizing faces', *British Journal of Psychology*, 1975, *66*, 409–26.

FENSTERHEIM, H. and TRESSELT, M. (1953), 'The influence of value systems on the perception of people', *Journal of Abnormal and Social Psychology*, *1*, 93–8.

FISHER, G. and COX, R. (1975), 'Recognizing human faces', *Applied Ergonomics*, *6*, 104–9.

FITZGIBBONS, D., GOLDBERG, L. and EAGLE, M. (1965), 'Field dependence and memory for incidental material', *Perceptual and Motor Skills*, *21*, 743–9.

FLEISHMAN, J., BUCKLEY, M., KLOSINSKY, M., SMITH, N. and TUCK, B. (1976), 'Judged attractiveness in recognition memory of women's faces', *Perceptual and Motor Skills*, *43*, 709–10.

FRANK, J. and FRANK, B. (1957), *Not Guilty*, Gollancz, London.

FREEDMAN, J. and HABER, R. (1974), 'One reason why we rarely forget a face', *Bulletin of Psychonomic Science*, *3*, 107–9.

FREUD, S. (1906), 'Psycho-analysis and the ascertaining of truth in courts of law', in *Collected Papers*, vol. 2, pp. 13–24, Basic Books, New York.

226

FREY, S. and von CRANACH, M. (1973), 'A method for the assessment of body movement variability', in M. von Cranach and I. Vine (eds), *Social Communication and Movement*, Academic Press, London and New York.

FRIEDMAN, M., REED, S. and CARTERETTE, E. (1971), 'Feature saliency and recognition memory for schematic faces', *Perception and Psychophysics*, *10*, 47–50.

FRIJDA, N. and VAN DE GEER, J. (1961), 'Codability and recognition: an experiment with facial expressions', *Acta Psychologica*, *18*, 360–7.

FURST, C., FULD, K. and PANCOE, M. (1974), 'Recall accuracy of eidetikers', *Journal of Experimental Psychology*, *102*, 1133–5.

GAHAGAN, L. (1933), 'Judgements of occupations from printed photographs', *Journal of Social Psychology*, *4*, 128–34.

GALE, A., MORRIS, P., LUCAS, B. and RICHARDSON, A. (1972), 'Types of imagery and imagery tapes: an EEG study', *British Journal of Psychology*, *63*, 523–31.

GALPER, R. (1970), 'Recognition of faces in photographic negative', *Psychonomic Science*, *19*, 207–8.

GALPER, R. (1973), '"Functional Race Membership" and recognition of faces', *Perceptual Motor Skills*, *37*, 455–62.

GALPER, R. and HOCHBERG, H. (1971), 'Recognition memory for photographs of faces', *American Journal of Psychology*, *84*, 351–4.

GARAI, J. and SCHEINFELD, A. (1968), 'Sex differences in mental and behavioural traits', *Genetic Psychology Monographs*, *77*, 169–299.

GARDNER, D. (1933), 'The perception and memory of witnesses', *Cornell Law Quarterly*, *18*, 391–409.

GARDNER, R. and LONG, R. (1960), 'The stability of cognitive controls', *Journal of Abnormal and Social Psychology*, *61*, 485–7.

GARDNER, R. and MORIARTY, A. (1968), *Personality Development at Preadolescence*, University of Washington Press, Seattle.

GARRETT, J. and KENNEDY, K. W. (1971), 'Collation of Anthropometry: II', *USAF AMRL Technical Report*, no. 68.

GARTON, R. and ALLEN, L. (1972), 'Recognition memory of paced and unpaced decision time for rare and common verbal material', *Perceptual and Motor Skills*, *35*, 548–50.

GIBSON, E. (1969), *Principles of Perceptual Learning and Development*, Appleton-Century-Crofts, New York.

GILBERT, C. and BAKAN, P. (1973), 'Visual asymmetry in perception of faces', *Neuropsychologia*, *11*, 355–62.

GILLILAND, A. and BURKE, R. (1926), 'A measure of sociability', *Journal of Applied Psychology*, *10*, 315–26.

GLANZER, M. and CLARK, W. (1964), 'The verbal loop hypothesis', *American Journal of Psychology*, *77*, 237–47.

GLONING, I., GLONING, K., HOFF, H. and TSCHABITSCHER, H. (1966), 'Zur Prosopagnosie', *Neuropsychology*, *4*, 113–31.

GOFFMAN, E. (1963), *Stigma: Notes on the management of spoiled identity*, Prentice-Hall, Englewood Cliffs.

GOLDSTEIN, A. (1965), 'Learning of inverted and normally oriented faces in children and adults *Psychonomic Science, 3*, 447–8.

GOLDSTEIN, A. (1975a), 'Eyewitness identification: a psychologist's view', Paper presented at American Psychology – Law Society, Chicago.

GOLDSTEIN, A. (1975b), 'Implications of differential face recognition data', Paper presented at the Midwestern Psychological Association Symposium, Chicago on Faces: How do we Perceive and Remember Them?

GOLDSTEIN, A. (1976), 'The fallibility of the eyewitness: psychological evidence', in B. D. Sales (ed.), *Psychology in the Legal Process*, Prentice-Hall, Englewood Cliffs.

GOLDSTEIN, A. (in press), *Eyewitness Identification : A Psychologist's View*,

GOLDSTEIN, A. and CHANCE, J. (1964), 'Recognition of children's faces', *Child Development, 35*, 129–36.

GOLDSTEIN, A. and CHANCE, J. (1971), 'Visual recognition memory for complex configurations', *Perception and Psychophysics, 9*, 237–41.

GOLDSTEIN, A. and CHANCE, J. (1974), 'Some factors in picture recognition memory', *Journal of General Psychology, 90*, 69–85.

GOLDSTEIN, A. and CHANCE, J. (1976), 'Measuring psychological similarity of faces', *Bulletin of the Psychonomic Society, 7*, 407–8.

GOLDSTEIN, A., HARMON, L. and LESK, A. (1971), 'Identification of human faces', *Proceedings of the IEEE, 59*, 748–60.

GOLDSTEIN, A., HARMON, L. and LESK, A. (1972), 'Man-machine interaction in human-face identification', *The Bell System Technical Journal, 51*, 399–427.

GOLDSTEIN, A. and MACKENBERG, E. (1966), 'Recognition of human faces from isolated feature: a developmental study', *Psychonomic Science, 6*, 149–50.

GRAY, C. and GUMMERMAN, K. (1975), 'The enigmatic eidetic image: a critical examination of method data and theories', *Psychological Bulletin, 82*, 383–407.

GREENE, H. (1975), 'Voiceprint identification: the case in favour of admissibility', *American Criminal Law Review, 13*, 171–200.

GREGORY, R. (1974), *Concepts and Mechanisms of Perception*, Duckworth, London.

GROPPER, G. (1963), 'Why is a picture worth a thousand words?' *Audio Visual Communication Review, 11*, 75–95.

GROSS, H. (1911), *Criminal Psychology*, 4th edition (M. Kallen translation), Paterson Smith, Mount Claire, New Jersey.

GUMMERMAN, K., GRAY, C. and WILSON, J. (1972), 'An attempt to assess eidetic imagery objectively', *Psychonomic Science, 28*, 115–18.

HAAF, R. (1974), 'Complexity and facial resemblance as determiners of response to face like stimuli by 5 and 10 week old infants', *Journal of Experimental Child Psychology, 18*, 480–7.

HAAF, R. and BROWN, C. (1976), 'Infants response to facelike patterns: Developmental changes between 10 and 15 weeks of age', *Journal of Experimental Child Psychology, 22*, 155–60.

HABER, R. (1969), 'Eidetic images', *Scientific American, 220,* 36–44.

HABER, R. and HABER, R. (1964), 'Eidetic imagery: I. frequency', *Perceptual and Motor Skills, 19,* 131–8.

HALL, E., MOUTON, J. and BLAKE, R. (1963), 'Group problem solving effectiveness under conditions of pooling vs. interaction', *Journal of Social Psychology, 59,* 147–57.

HALL, M. (1974), 'The current status of speaker identification by use of speech spectrograms', *Canadian Journal of Forensic Science, 7,* 152–76.

HANAWALT, N. and DEMAREST, I. (1939), 'The effects of verbal suggestion in the recall period upon the reproduction of visually perceived forms', *Journal of Experimental Psychology, 25,* 159–74.

HARGREAVES, W. and STARKWEATHER, J. (1963), 'Recognition of speaker identity', *Language and Speech, 6,* 63–7.

HARMON, L. (1973), 'The recognition of faces', *Scientific American, 229,* 71–83.

HARMON, L. and JULESZ, B. (1973), 'Masking in visual recognition', *Science, 180,* 1194–7.

HARMON, L. and MURRAY-HILL, N. (1971), 'Some aspects of recognition of human faces', in O. Gruesser (ed.), *Pattern Recognition in Biological and Technical Systems,* Springer-Verlag, New York.

HARRIS, C. and HABER, R. (1963), 'Selective attention and coding in visual perception', *Journal of Experimental Psychology, 65,* 328–33.

HARRIS, R. (1973), 'Answering questions containing marked and unmarked adjectives and adverbs', *Journal of Experimental Psychology, 97,* 399–401.

HASTORF, A. and CANTRILL, H. (1954), 'They saw a game: a case study', *Journal of Abnormal and Social Psychology, 49,* 129–234.

HEBB, D. and FOORD, E. (1945), 'Errors of visual recognition and the nature of the trace', *Journal of Experimental Psychology, 35,* 335–48.

HECAEN, H. and ANGELERGUES, R. (1962), 'Agnosia for faces (prosopagnosia)', *Archives of Neurology, 7,* 92–100.

HECKER, M. (1971), 'Speaker recognition', *American Speech and Hearing Association,* monograph no. 16.

HECKER, M., STEVENS, K., VON BISMARCK, G. and WILLIAMS, C. (1968), 'Manifestations of task-induced stress in the acoustic speech signal', *Journal of the Acoustical Society of America, 44,* 993.

HENNESSY, J. and ROMIG, C. (1971), 'A review of the experiments involving voiceprint identification', *Journal of Forensic Science, 16,* 183–98.

HEWES, G. (1957), 'The anthropology of posture', *Scientific American, 196,* 123–32.

HOCHBERG, J. (1964), *Perception,* Prentice-Hall, Englewood Cliffs.

HOCHBERG, J. and GALPER, R. (1967), 'Recognition of faces (1). An exploratory study', *Psychonomic Science, 12,* 619–20.

HOCHBERG, J. and GALPER, R. (1974), 'Attribution of intention as a function of physiognomy', *Memory and Cognition, 2,* 39–42.

HOFFMAN, C. and KAGAN, S. (1977), 'Field dependence and facial recognition', *Perceptual and Motor Skills, 44,* 119–24.

Bibliography

HOLLEIN, H. and MCGLONE, R. (1976), 'An evaluation of the voiceprint technique of speaker identification', *Proceedings of the Garnahan Crime Countermeasures Conference*, 39–45.

HOLZMAN, P. and GARDNER, R. (1960), 'Levelling and sharpening and memory organization', *Journal of Abnormal and Social Psychology*, *61*, 176–80.

HOMA, D., HAVER, B. and SCHWARTZ, T. (1976), 'Perceptibility of schematic face stimuli: evidence for a perceptual Gestalt', *Memory and Cognition*, *4*, 176–85.

HOPPER, W. (1973), 'Photofit', *Journal of the Forensic Science Society*, *13*, 77–82.

HOWELLS, T. (1938), 'A study of ability to recognize faces', *Journal of Abnormal and Social Psychology*, *33*, 124–7.

HUCKABEE, M. (1974), 'Introversion – extroversion and imagery', *Psychological Reports*, *34*, 453–4.

HULL, C. (1928), *Aptitude Testing*, Harrap, New York.

HUNT, T. (1928), 'The measurement of social intelligence', *Journal of Applied Psychology*, *12*, 317–33.

HUNTER, I. (1964), *Memory*, Penguin Books, Harmondsworth.

HURWITZ, D., WIGGINS, N. and JONES, L. (1975), 'Semantic differential for facial attributions: the face differential', *Bulletin of the Psychonomic Society*, *6*, 370–2.

HUTCHINS, R. and SLESINGER, D. (1928), 'Some observations on the law of evidence: spontaneous exclamations', *Columbia Law Review*, *28*, 432.

HUTT, C. (1972), *Males and Females*, Penguin Books, Harmondsworth.

JAENSCH, E. (1930), *Eidetic Imagery and Topological Methods of Investigation* (O. Oeser translation), Kegan Paul, Trench, Trubner, London (Harcourt Brace, New York).

JENKINS, J. (1974), 'Can we have a theory of meaningful memory?' in R. Solso (ed.), *Theories in Cognitive Psychology*, Lawrence Erlbaum Associates, Potomac, Maryland.

JENKINS, J., STACK, W. and DENO, S. (1969), 'Children's recognition and recall of picture and word stimuli', *Audio Visual Communication Review*, *17*, 265–71.

JONES, F. and HANSON, J. (1961), 'Time-space pattern in a gross body movement,' *Perceptual and Motor Skills*, *12*, 35–41.

JONES, F. and HANSON, J. (1962), 'Note on the persistence of pattern in a gross movement', *Perceptual and Motor Skills*, *14*, 230.

JONES, L. and HIRSCHBERG, N. (1975), 'What's in a face? Individual differences in facial perception', Paper presented at the 83rd Annual Convention of the American Psychological Association.

KAGAN, J. and HAVEMANN, E. (1972), *Psychology: An Introduction*, 2nd edition, Harcourt Brace Jovanovich, New York.

KAY, H. (1955), 'Learning and retaining verbal material', *British Journal of Psychology*, *46*, 81–100.

KAY, H. and SKEMP, R. (1956), 'Differential thresholds for recognition – further experiments on interpolated recall and recognition', *Quarterly Journal of Experimental Psychology*, *8*, 153–62.

KENDON, A. (1971), 'Some relationships between body motion and speech', in A. Siegman and B. Pope (eds), *Studies in Dyadic Communication*, Pergamon, London.

KERSTA, L. (1962), 'Voiceprint identification', *Nature, 196,* 1253-7.

KIESLER, C. (1971), *The Psychology of Commitment,* Academic Press, New York and London.

KING, D. (1971), 'The use of photo-fit 1970-1971, a progress report', *Police Research Bulletin, 18,* 40-4.

KINTSCH, W. (1970), 'Models for free recall and recognition', in D. Norman (ed.), *Models of Human Memory,* Academic Press, New York and London.

KLEINSMITH, L. and KAPLAN, S. (1963), 'Paired associate learning as a function of arousal and interpolated interval', *Journal of Experimental Psychology, 65,* 190-3.

KLINE, P. (1972), *Fact and Fantasy in Freudian Theory,* Methuen, London.

KLUVER, H. (1931), 'The eidetic child', in C. Murchison (ed.), *A Handbook of Child Psychology,* Clark University Press, Worcester, Mass.

KLUVER, H. (1932), 'Eidetic phenomena', *Psychological Bulletin, 29,* 181-203.

KNAPP, M. (1972), *Non-verbal Communication in Human Interaction,* Holt, Rinehart and Winston, New York.

KOBLER, G. (1915), cited in G. Whipple, 'Psychology of testimony', *Psychological Bulletin, 12,* 221-4.

KOGAN, N. (1970), 'Educational aspects of cognitive style', in G. Lessor (ed.), *Psychology and Educational Practice,* Scott Foresman, London.

KOGAN, N., STEVENS, J. and SHELTON, F. (1961), 'Age differences: a developmental study of discriminability and affective response', *Journal of Abnormal and Social Psychology, 62,* 221-30.

KOHLER, I. (1962), 'Experiments with goggles', *Scientic Afimerican, 206,* 62-72.

KONORSKI, J. (1967), *Integrative Activity of the Brain,* University of Chicago Press.

KOULACK, D. and TUTHILL, J. (1972), 'Height perception: a function of social distance', *Canadian Journal of Behavioural Science, 4,* 50-3.

KOZENY, E. (1962), 'Experimentelle Untersuchungen zur Ausdruckskunde mittel photographisch-statistischer Methode' (Experimental investigation of physiognomy utilizing a photographic-statistical method), *Archiv für die Gesamte Psychologie, 114,* 55-71.

KRAMER, E. (1963), 'Judgement of personal characteristics and emotions from nonverbal properties of speech', *Psychological Bulletin, 6,* 408-20.

KREEZER, G. and GLANVILLE, A. (1937), 'A method for the quantitative analysis of human gait', *Journal of Genetic Psychology, 50,* 109-36.

KRETSCHMER, E. (1936), *Physique and Character,* Cooper Square, New York.

Bibliography

KUBIE, L. (1959), 'Implications for legal procedure of the fallibility of human memory', *University of Pasadena Law Review, 108*, 59.

KUEHN, L. (1974), 'Looking down a gun barrel: person perception and violent crime', *Perceptual and Motor Skills, 39*, 1159–64.

KURTZ, K. and HOVLAND, C. (1953), 'The effect of verbalization during observation of stimulus objects upon accuracy of recognition and recall', *Journal of Experimental Psychology, 45*, 157–64.

LADGEFOGED, P. and VANDERSLICE, R. (1967), 'The voiceprint mystique', *Working Papers in Phonetics, 7*, University of California.

LANDAUER, T. (1972), *'Psychology: a Brief Overview'*, McGraw-Hill, New York.

LANDIS, E. and PHELPS, L. (1928), 'The prediction from photographs of success and of vocational aptitude', *Journal of Experimental Psychology, 3*, 313–24.

LANDY, D. and ARONSON, E. (1969), 'The influence of the character of the criminal and his victim on the decisions of simulated jurors', *Journal of Experimental Social Psychology, 5*, 141–52.

LAUGHERY, K., cited in A. Goldstein (in press), *'Eyewitness Identification: A Psychologist's View'*.

LAUGHERY, K., ALEXANDER, J. and LANE, A. (1971), 'Recognition of human faces: effects of target exposure, target position, pose position and type of photograph', *Journal of Applied Psychology, 55*, 477–83.

LAUGHERY, K., FESSLER, P., LENOROVITZ, D. and YOBLICK, D. (1974), 'Time delay and similarity effects in facial recognition', *Journal of Applied Psychology, 49*, 490–6.

LAVRAKAS, P., BURI, J. and MAYZNER, M. (1976), 'A perspective on the recognition of other-race faces', *Perception and Psychophysics, 20*, 475–81.

LEASK, J., HABER, R. and HABER, R. (1969), 'Eidetic imagery in children: 11. longitudinal and experimental results', *Psychonomic Monograph Supplements, 3*, (3, whole no. 35).

LERNER, R. and KORN, S. (1972), 'The development of body-build stereotypes in males', *Child Development, 43*, 908–20.

LERNER, R. and MOORE, T. (1974), 'Sex and status effects on the perception of physical attractiveness', *Psychological Reports, 34*, 1047–50.

LEVINE, F. and TAPP, J. (1971), cited in F. Levine and J. Tapp, 'The psychology of criminal identification: the gap from Wade to Kirby', *University of Pennsylvania Law Review, 121*, 1079–132.

LEVINE, F. and TAPP, J. (1973), 'The psychology of criminal identification: the gap from Wade to Kirby', *University of Pennsylvania Law Review, 121*, 1079–132.

LEVY, A. and HESHKA, A. (1973), 'Similarity and the false recognition of prototypes', *Bulletin of the Psychonomic Society, 1*, 181–2.

LIGGETT, J. (1974), *The Human Face*, Constable, London.

LINDZEY, G., PRINCE, B. and WRIGHT, W. (1952), 'A study of facial asymmetry', *Journal of Personality, 21*, 68–84.

232

LINTON, H. (1955), 'Dependence on external influence: correlates in perception, attitudes and judgements', *Journal of Abnormal and Social Psychology, 51,* 502–7.

LITTERER, O. (1933), 'Stereotypes', *Journal of Social Psychology, 4,*59–68.

LITTMAN, R. (1961), 'Psychology. The socially indifferent science', *American Psychologist, 16,* 232.

LOFTUS, E. (1974), 'Reconstructing memory: the incredible eyewitness', *Psychology Today, 8,* 116–19.

LOFTUS, E. (1975), 'Leading questions and the eyewitness report', *Cognitive Psychology, 7,* 560–72.

LOFTUS, E., ALTMAN, D. and GEBALLE, R. (1975), 'Effects of questioning upon a witness's later recollections', *Journal of Police Science and Administration, 3,* 162–5.

LOFTUS, E. and PALMER, J. (1974), 'Reconstruction of automobile destruction: an example of the interaction between language and memory', *Journal of Verbal Learning and Verbal Behaviour, 13,* 585–9.

LOFTUS, E. and ZANNI, G. (1975), 'Eyewitness testimony: the influence of the wording of a question', *Bulletin of the Psychonomic Society, 5,* 86–8.

LUCE, T. (1974), 'Blacks, white and yellows: they all look alike to me', *Psychology Today, 8,* 107–8.

LYKKEN, D. (1974), 'Psychology and the lie detector industry', *American Psychologist, 29,* 725–39.

MCCALL, G., MAZANEC, N., ERIKSON, W. and SMITH, H. (1974), 'Same-sex recall effects in tests of observational accuracy', *Perceptual and Motor Skills, 36,* 830.

MCCARTY, D. (1929), *Psychology for the Lawyer,* Prentice-Hall, Englewood Cliffs.

MCCURDY, H. (1949), 'Experimental notes on the asymmetry of the human face', *Journal of Abnormal and Social Psychology, 44,* 553–5.

MCGEHEE, F. (1937), 'The reliability of the identification of the human voice', *Journal of General Psychology, 17,* 249–71.

MACGREGOR, F., ABEL, T., BRYT, A., LAUER, E. and WEISSMANN, S. (1953), *Facial Deformities and Plastic Surgery,* C. C. Thomas, Springfield, Illinois.

MCKELLAR, P. (1972), 'Imagery from the standpoint of introspection', in P. Sheehan (ed.), *The Function and Nature of Imagery,* Academic Press, London and New York.

MCKELVIE, S. (1972), 'Strategies of encoding in memory for faces', PhD thesis, McGill University.

MCKELVIE, S. (1973), 'The meaningfulness and meaning of schematic faces', *Perception and Psychophysics, 14,* 343–8.

MCKELVIE, S. (1976a), 'The role of eyes and mouth in recognition memory for faces', *American Journal of Psychology, 89,* 311–23.

MCKELVIE, S. (1976b), 'The effect of verbal labelling on recognition memory for schematic faces', *Quarterly Journal of Experimental Psychology, 28,* 459–74.

Bibliography

MALPASS, R. and KRAVITZ, J. (1969), 'Recognition for faces of own and other "race"', *Journal of Personality and Social Psychology, 13,* 330–5.

MALPASS, R., LAVIGUEUR, H. and WELDON, D. (1973), 'Verbal and visual training in face recognition', *Perception and Psychophysics, 14,* 285–92.

MANDLER, G. (1972), 'Organization and recognition', in E. Tulving and W. Donaldson (eds), *Organisation of Memory,* Academic Press, New York and London.

MANDLER, J. and JOHNSON, N. (1976), 'Some of the thousand words a picture is worth', *Journal of Experimental Psychology: Human Learning and Memory, 2,* 529–40.

MANDLER, J. and PARKER, R. (1976), 'Memory for descriptive and spatial information in complex pictures', *Journal of Experimental Psychology: Human Learning and Memory, 2,* 38-48.

MANDLER, J. and STEIN, N. (1974), 'Recall and recognition of pictures by children as a function of organization and distractor similarity', *Journal of Experimental Psychology, 102,* 657–69.

MARKS, D. (1972), 'Individual differences in the vividness of visual imagery and their effects on function', in P. W. Sheehan (ed.), *The Function and Nature of Imagery,* Academic Press, London and New York.

MARKS, E. (1943), 'Skin colour judgements of negro college students', *Journal of Abnormal and Social Psychology, 38,* 370–6.

MARQUIS, K., MARSHALL, J. and OSKAMP, S. (1972), 'Testimony validity as a function of question form, atmosphere, and item difficulty', *Journal of Applied Social Psychology, 2,* 167–86.

MARSH, J. and ABBOT, H. (1945), 'An investigation of after-images', *Journal of Comparative Psychology, 38,* 47–63.

MARSHALL, J. (1966), *Law and Psychology in Conflict,* Anchor Books, New York.

MARSHALL, J. (1969), 'The evidence: Do we see and hear what is? Or do our senses lie?', *Psychology Today, 2,* 49–52.

MARSHALL, J. and HANSSEN, E. cited in *Sunday Times,* 'The selective memory' (Spectrum), 19 May 1974.

MARSTON, W. (1924), 'Studies in testimony', *Journal of the American Institute of Criminal Law, 15,* 5–31.

MARTIN, T. (1974), 'Application of limited vocabulary recognition systems', in D. Redd (ed.), *Speech Recognition,* Academic Press, New York and London.

MASLOW, A. (1946), 'Problem-centering vs. means-centering in science', *Philosophy of Science, 13,* 326–31.

MAZANEC, N. and MCCALL, G. (1975), 'Sex, cognitive categories and observational accuracy', *Psychological Reports, 37,* 987–90.

MEENES, M. and MORTON, M. (1936), 'Characteristics of the eidetic phenomena', *Journal of General Psychology, 14,* 370–91.

MESSICK, S. (1970), 'The criterion problem in the evaluation of instruction: assessing possible, not just intended, outcomes', in M. Wittrock and D. Wiley (eds), *The Evaluation of Instruction: Issues and Problems*, Holt, Rinehart & Winston, New York.

MESSICK, S. and DAMARIN, F. (1964), 'Cognitive styles and memory for faces', *Journal of Abnormal and Social Psychology*, 69, 313–18.

MILLER, D. and LOFTUS, E. (1976), 'Influencing memory for people and their actions', *Bulletin of the Psychonomic Society*, 7, 9–11.

MILLER, N. and DOLLARD, J. (1941), *Social Learning and Imitation*, Yale University Press, New Haven.

MILNER, B. (1968), 'Visual recognition and recall after right temporal lobe excision in man', *Neuropsychologia*, 6, 191–209.

MONAHAN, F. (1941), *Women in Crime*, Ives Washburn, New York.

MORRIS, P. and GALE, A. (1974), 'A correlational study of variables related to imagery', *Perceptual and Motor Skills*, 38, 659–65.

MORTON, D. and FULLER, D. (1952), *Human Locomotion and Body Form*, Williams & Wilkins, New York.

MUNSTERBERG, H. (1908), *On the witness stand: Essays on Psychology and Crime*, Clark, Boardman, New York.

MULAC, A., HANLEY, T. and PRIGGE, D. (1974), 'Effects of phonological speech foreignness upon three dimensions of attitude of selected American listeners', *Quarterly Journal of Speech*, 60, 411–20.

MUNN, N. (1961), *Psychology: The Fundamentals of Human Adjustment*, Harrap, New York.

MURDOCH, B. (1968), 'Modality effects in short term memory: storage or retrieval', *Journal of Experimental Psychology*, 77, 79–86.

MURRAY, H. (1938), *Explorations in Personality*, Oxford University Press, New York.

MURRAY, T. and CORT, S. (1971), 'Aural identification of children's voices', *Journal of Auditory Research*, 11, 260–2.

MUSCIO, B. (1915), 'The influence of the form of the question', *British Journal of Psychology*, 8, 351–89.

NASH, H. (1969), 'Recognition of body surface regions', *Genetic Psychology Monographs*, 79, 297–340.

NATIONAL COUNCIL FOR CIVIL LIBERTIES (1974), *Memorandum of Evidence to the Devlin Committee on Identification Parades and Procedures*, London.

NEISSER, U. (1967), *Cognitive Psychology*, Appleton-Century-Crofts, New York.

NELSON, D. and BROOKS, D. (1973), 'Functional independence of pictures and their verbal memory codes', *Journal of Experimental Psychology*, 98, 44–8.

NELSON, D. and REED, V. (1976), 'On the nature of pictorial encoding: a levels of processing analysis', *Journal of Experimental Psychology: Human Learning and Memory*, 2, 49–57.

NELSON, T. (1968), 'The effects of training in attention deployment on observing behaviour in reflective and impulsive children', unpublished doctoral dissertation, University of Minnesota.

Bibliography

NICKERSON, R. (1965), 'Short term memory for complex, meaningful visual configurations: a demonstration of capacity', *Canadian Journal of Psychology*, *19*, 155–60.

NIELSEN, G. and SMITH, E. (1973), 'Imaginal and verbal representations in short-term recognition of visual forms', *Journal of Experimental Psychology*, *101*, 375–8.

NORMAN, D. (1968), 'Towards a theory of memory and attention', *Psychological Review*, *75*, 522–36.

NOTON, D. and STARK, L. (1971), 'Scan paths in eye movements during pattern perception', *Science*, *171*, 308–11.

OBSERVER (1975), article on George Davis' case, 11 May.

ORNE, M. (1962), 'On the social psychology of the psychology experiment', *American Psychologist*, *17*, 776–83.

OTIS, M. (1924), 'A study of suggestibility of children', *Archives of Psychology*, no. 70.

PAIVIO, A. (1969), 'Mental imagery in associative learning and memory', *Psychological Review*, *76*, 241–63.

PAIVIO, A. (1971), *Imagery and Verbal Processes*, Holt, Rinehart Winston, New York.

PAIVIO, A. (1976), 'Imagery in recall and recognition', in J. Brown (ed.), *Recall and Recognition*, Wiley, New York.

PENRY, J. (1971), *Looking at Faces and Remembering Them*, Elek Books, London.

PETERS, A. (1917), cited in H. Ellis, 'Recognizing faces', *British Journal of Psychology*, 1975, *66*, 409–26.

POLLACK, I., PICKETT, J. and SUMBY, W. (1954), 'On the identification of speakers by voice', *Journal of the Acoustical Society of America*, *26*, 403–6.

POSTMAN, L. (1972), 'A pragmatic view of organisation theory', in E. Tulving and W. Donaldson (eds), *Organisation of Memory*, Academic Press, New York and London.

POSTMAN, L. (1976), 'Interference theory revisited', in J. Brown (ed.), *Recall and Recognition*, Wiley, New York.

POTTER, M. (1976), 'Short term conceptual memory for pictures', *Journal of Experimental Psychology: Human Learning and Memory*, *2*, 509–22.

POTTER, M. and LEVY, E. (1969), 'Recognition memory for a rapid sequence of pictures', *Journal of Experimental Psychology*, *81*, 10–15.

POWELL, G., TUTTON, S. and STEWART, R. (1974), 'The differential stereotyping of similar physiques', *British Journal of Social and Clinical Psychology*, *13*, 421–3.

POWIS, D. (1974), A booklet 'Thieves on Wheels' cited in Peter Evans, *The Police Revolution*, Allen & Unwin, London.

PRENTICE, W. (1954), 'Visual recognition of verbally labelled figures', *American Journal of Psychology*, *67*, 315–20.

PROST, J. (1965), 'The methodology of gait analysis and gaits of monkeys', *American Journal of Physiological Anthropology*, *23*, 215–40.

PTACEK, P. and SANDERS, E. (1966), 'Age recognition from voice', *Journal of Speech and Hearing Research, 9,* 273–7.

PYLYSHYN, Z. (1973), 'What the minds eye tells the minds brain: A critique of mental imagery', *Psychological Bulletin, 80,* 1–24.

RAZRAN, G. (1938), 'Conditioning away social bias by the luncheon technique', *Psychological Bulletin, 35,* 693.

RAZRAN, G. (1950), 'Ethnic dislikes and stereotypes', *Journal of Abnormal and Social Psychology, 45,* 7–27.

REICHER, G. (1969), 'Perceptual recognition as a function of meaningfulness of stimulus material', *Journal of Experimental Psychology, 81,* 275–80.

REIFF, R. and SCHEERER, M. (1959), *Memory and Hypnotic Age Regression,* International University Press, New York.

RESTLE, F. (1974), 'Critique of pure memory', in R. Solso (ed.), *Theories in Cognitive Psychology,* Lawrence Erbaum Associates, Potomac, Maryland.

RICH, J. (1975), 'Effects of children's physical attractiveness on teachers' evaluations', *Journal of Educational Psychology, 67,* 599–609.

RICHARDSON, A. (1969), *Mental Imagery,* Springer, New York.

RILEY, D. (1962), 'Memory for form', in L. Postman (ed.), *Psychology in the Making,* Knoft, New York.

RINGEL, W. (1968), *Identification and Police Line-ups,* Gould, New York.

ROCK, I. (1974), 'The perception of distorted figures', *Scientific American, 230,* 78–85.

ROLL, S. and VERINIS, J. (1971), 'Stereotypes of scalp and facial hair as measured by the semantic differential', *Psychological Reports, 28,* 975–80.

ROLPH, C. (1957), *Personal Identity,* Thomas, New York.

ROSENTHAL, R. (1966), *Experimenter Effects in Behavioural Research,* Appleton-Century-Crofts, New York.

RUMP, E. and DELIN, P. (1973), 'Differential accuracy of the status-height phenomenon and an experimenter effect', *Journal of Personality and Social Psychology, 28,* 343–7.

RUPP, A., WARMBRAND, A., KARASH, A. and BUCKHOUT, R. (1976), 'Effects of group interaction of eyewitness reports', Paper presented at the meeting of the Eastern Psychological Association, New York.

SACHS, J. (1967), 'Recognition memory for syntactic and semantic aspects of connected discourse', *Perception and Psychophysics, 2,* 437–42.

SACHS, J. (1974), 'Memory in reading and listening to discourse', *Memory and Cognition, 2,* 95–100.

SAKAI, T., NAGAO, M. and KANADE, T. (1972), 'Computer analysis and classification of human faces', *First USA-Japan Computer Conference Proceedings.*

SALAPATEK, P. and KESSON, W. (1966), 'Visual scanning of triangles by the human newborn', *Journal of Experimental Child Psychology, 3,* 155–67.

SALTHOUSE, T. (1974), 'Using selective interference to investigate spatial memory representations', *Memory and Cognition, 2,* 749–57.

Bibliography

SAMPSON, J. (1970), 'Free recall of verbal and non-verbal stimuli', *Quarterly Journal of Experimental Psychology*, *22*, 215–21.

SAMUELS, M. R. (1939), 'Judgements of faces', *Character and Personality*, *8*, 18–27.

SANTA, J. and BAKER, L. (1975), 'Linguistic influences on visual memory', *Memory and Cognition*, *3*, 445–50.

SANTA, J. and RANKEN, H. (1972), 'Effects of verbal coding on recognition memory', *Journal of Experimental Psychology*, *93*, 268–78.

SCAPINELLO, K. and YARMEY, D. (1970), 'The role of familiarity and orientation in immediate and delayed recognition of pictorial stimuli', *Psychonomic Science*, *21*, 329–30.

SCHERER, K. (1974), 'Voice quality analysis of American and German speakers', *Journal of Psycholinguistic Research*, *3*, 281–98.

SCHILL, T. (1966), 'Effects of approval motivation and varying conditions of verbal reinforcement on incidental memory for faces', *Psychological Reports*, *19*, 55–60.

SECORD, P. (1958), 'Facial features and inference processes in interpersonal perception', R. Tagiuri and L. Petrullo (eds), *Person Perception and Interpersonal Behaviour*, Stanford University Press.

SECORD, P., BEVAN, W. and KATZ, B. (1956), 'The negro stereotype and perceptual accentuation', *Journal of Abnormal and Social Psychology*, *53*, 78–83.

SECORD, P., DUKES, W. and BEVAN, W. (1954), 'Personalities in faces: I. An experiment in social perceiving', *Genetic Psychology Monographs*, *49*, 231–79.

SHAPIRO, J. (1968), 'Responsibility to facial and linguistic cues', *Journal of Communication*, *18*, 11–17.

SHEEHAN, P. (1966), 'Accuracy and vividness of visual images', *Perceptual and Motor Skills*, *23*, 391–9.

SHEEHAN, P. (1967), 'Visual imagery and the organisational properties of perceived stimuli', *British Journal of Psychology*, *58*, 247–52.

SHEEHAN, P. and NEISSER, U. (1969), 'Some variables affecting the vividness of imagery in recall', *British Journal of Psychology*, *60*, 71–80.

SHELDON, W. and STEVENS, S. (1942), *The Varieties of Temperament*, Harper & Row, New York.

SHEPARD, R. (1967), 'Recognition memory for words, sentences and pictures', *Journal of Verbal Learning and Verbal Behaviour*, *6*, 156–63.

SHEPHERD, J., DEREGOWSKI, J. and ELLIS, H. D. (1974), 'A cross-cultural study of recognition memory for faces', *International Journal of Psychology*, *9*, 205–11.

SHEPHERD, J. and ELLIS, H. D. (1973), 'The effect of attractiveness on recognition memory for faces', *American Journal of Psychology*, *86*, 627–33.

SHIPP, T. and HOLLEIN, H. (1969), 'Perception of the aging male voice', *Journal of Speech and Hearing Research*, *12*, 703–10.

SHOEMAKER, D., SOUTH, D. and LOWE, J. (1973), 'Facial stereotypes of deviants and judgements of guilt or innocence', *Social Forces*, *51*, 427–33.

238

SIGALL, H. and OSTROVE, N. (1974), 'The effect of the physical attractiveness of the defendant and nature of the crime on juridic judgement', Paper presented at the 81st Annual Convention of the American Psychological Association.

SIMMONDS, D., POULTON, E. and TICKNER, A. (1975), 'Identifying people in a videotape recording made at night', *Ergonomics, 18*, 607–18.

SLOBIN, D. (1971), *Psycholinguistics*, Scott, Foresman, New York.

SMITH, E. and NIELSEN, G. (1970), 'Representations and retrieval processes in STM recognition and recall of faces', *Journal of Experimental Psychology, 85*, 397–405.

SMITH, H. (1966), *Sensitivity to People*, McGraw-Hill, New York.

SNEE, T. and LUSH, D. (1941), 'Interaction of the narrative and interrogatory methods of obtaining testimony', *Journal of Psychology, 11*, 229–330.

SORCE, J. and CAMPOS, J. (1974), 'The role of expression in the recognition of a face', *American Journal of Psychology, 87*, 71–82.

SPERLING, G. (1960), 'The information available in brief visual presentations', *Psychological Monographs, 74*, whole no. 498.

SPERLING, G. (1967), 'Successive approximations to a model of short-term memory', *Acta Psychologica, 27*, 285–92.

STAFFIERI, R. (1972), 'Body build and behavioural expectancies in young females', *Developmental Psychology, 6*, 125–7.

STANDING, L. (1973), 'Learning 10,000 pictures', *Quarterly Journal of Experimental Psychology, 25*, 207–22.

STANDING, L., CONEZIO, J. and HABER, R. (1970), 'Perception and memory for pictures: single trial learning of 2560 visual stimuli', *Psychonomic Science, 19*, 73–4.

STERN, L. W. (ed.) (1903–6), *Beitrage zur Psychologie der Aussage*, Leipzig.

STERN, L. W. (1910), 'Abstracts of lectures on the psychology of testimony and on the study of individuality', *American Journal of Psychology, 21*, 270–81.

STERN, L. W. (1924), *Psychology of Early Childhood*, Allen & Unwin, London.

STERN, L. W. (1938), *General Psychology from the Personalistic Standpoint*, Macmillan, New York.

STERN, L. W. (1939), 'The psychology of testimony', *Journal of Abnormal and Social Psychology, 34*, 3–20.

STEVENS, K., WILLIAMS, C., CARBONELL, J. and WOODS, B. (1968), 'Speaker authentication and identification: A comparison of spectrographic and auditory presentation of speech material', *Journal of the Acoustical Society of America, 44*, 1596–1607.

STRATTON, G. (1897), 'Vision without inversion of the retinal image', *Psychological Review, 4*, 341–60, 463–81.

STRITCH, T. and SECORD, P. (1956), 'Interaction effects in the perception of faces', *Journal of Personality, 24*, 272–84.

Bibliography

STROMEYER, C. (1970), 'The mnemonic feat of the "Shass Pollak"', *Psychological Review*, *24*, 244–7.

STROMEYER, C. and PSOTKA, J. (1970), 'The detailed texture of eidetic images', *Nature*, *225*, 346–9.

SUNDAY TIMES (1974), 'The selective memory', 19 May.

TAGIURI, R. and PETRULLO, L. (1958), *Person Perception and Interpersonal Behaviour*, Stanford University Press.

TERRY, R. L. and SNIDER, W. (1972), 'Veridicality of interpersonal perceptions based upon physiognomic cues', *Journal of Psychology*, *81*, 208.

THORNDYKE, P. (1976), 'The role of inferences in discourse comprehension', *Journal of Verbal Learning and Verbal Behaviour*, *15*, 437–46.

THORNTON, G. (1939), 'The ability to judge crimes from photographs of criminals', *Journal of Abnormal and Social Psychology*, *34*, 378–83.

THORNTON, G. (1943), 'The effect upon judgements of personality traits of varying a single factor in a photograph', *Journal of Social Psychology*, *18*, 127–48.

TICKNER, A. and POULTON, E. (1975), 'Watching for people and actions', *Ergonomics*, *18*, 35–51.

TOSI, O., OYER, W., LASHBROOK, C., PEDREY, J. and NASH, E. (1972), 'Experiment on voice identification', *Journal of the Acoustical Society of America*, *51*, 2030–43.

TRANKELL, A. (1972), *Reliability of Evidence*, Beckmans, Stockholm.

TRAXEL, W. (1962), 'Kritische Untersuchungen zur Eidetik', *Archiv für die Gesamte Psychologie*, *114*, 206–336.

TULVING, E. and THOMPSON, D. (1971), 'Retrieval processes in recognition memory: effects of associative context', *Journal of Experimental Psychology*, *87*, 116–24.

TULVING, E. and THOMPSON, D. (1973), 'Encoding specificity and retrieval processes in episodic memory', *Psychological Review*, *80*, 352–73.

TVERSKY, B. (1969), 'Similarity of schematic faces: a test of interdimensional additivity', *Perception and Psychophysics*, *5*, 124–7.

VERINIS, J. and WALKER, V. (1970), 'Policemen and the recall of criminal details', *Journal of Social Psychology*, *81*, 217–21.

WALKER, P. (1972), *Identification Parade*, Hale, London.

WALL, P. (1965), *Eyewitness Identification in Criminal Cases*, Thomas, New York.

WALLACE, G., COLTHEART, M. and FORSTER, K. (1970), 'Reminiscence in recognition memory for faces', *Psychonomic Science*, *18*, 335–6.

WALLACH, H. and AVERBACH, E. (1955), 'On memory modalities', *American Journal of Psychology*, *68*, 249–57.

WALLACH, M., KOGAN, N. and BURT, R. (1967), 'Group risk taking and field dependence-independence of group members', *Sociometry*, *30*, 323–38.

WALTER, G. (1953), *The Living Brain*, Norton, New York.

WANNER, E. (1974), *On Remembering, Forgetting and Understanding Sentences*, Mouton, The Hague and Paris.

WARR, P. (1973), 'Towards a more human psychology', *Bulletin of the British Psychological Society*, *26*, 1–8.

WARR, P. and KNAPPER, C. (1968), *The Perception of People and Events*, Wiley, Chichester.

WARREN COMMISSION REPORT (1964), Warren Commission Report on the Assassination of President Kennedy, ed. P. Ballot, Scanartronics Corporation, Island Park, New York.

WASSERMAN, J., WIGGINS, N., JONES, L. and ITKIN, S. (1974), 'A cross cultural study of the attribution of personological characteristics as a function of facial perception', *American Psychological Association Proceedings*, New Orleans.

WEBB, W. (1961), 'The choice of problem', *American Psychologist*, *16*, 223–7.

WELD, H. (1954), 'Legal psychology: the psychology of testimony', in F. Marcuse (ed.), *Areas of Psychology*, Harper, New York.

WHIPPLE, G. (1909), 'The observer as reporter: a survey of the "psychology of testimony"', *Psychological Bulletin*, *6*, 153–70.

WHIPPLE, G. (1910), 'Recent literature on the psychology of testimony', *Psychological Bulletin*, *7*, 365.

WHIPPLE, G. (1912), 'Psychology of testimony and report', *Psychological Bulletin*, *9*, 264–9.

WHIPPLE, G. (1917), 'Psychology of testimony', *Psychological Bulletin*, *14*, 234.

WHITELY, R. and MCGEOCH, J. (1927), 'The Effect of one form of report upon another', *American Journal of Psychology*, *38*, 280.

WICKENS, D. (1970), 'Encoding categories of words: an empirical approach to meaning', *Psychological Review*, *77*, 1–15.

WICKENS, D. (1972), 'Characteristics of word encoding', in A. Melton and E. Martin (eds), *Coding Processes in Human Memory*, Wiley, New York.

WILLIAMS, C. and STEVENS, K. (1969), 'On determining the emotional state of pilots during flight', *Aerospace Medicine*, *40*, 1369.

WILLIAMS, G. and HAMMELMANN, H. (1963), 'Identification parades', *Criminal Law Review*, *1*, 479–90.

WILLIAMS, L. (1975), 'Application of signal detection parameters in a test of eyewitnesses to a crime', Report no. CR–20, *Center for Responsive Psychology*, New York.

WILSON, G. and NIAS, D. (1976), *Love's Mysteries*, Open Books, London.

WILSON, J. (1975), *Thinking About Crime*, Basic Books, New York.

WILSON, P. (1968), 'Perceptual distortion of height as a function of ascribed academic status', *Journal of Social Psychology*, *74*, 97–102.

WITKIN, H., DYK, R., FATERSON, H., GOODENOUGH, D. and KARP, S. (1962), *Psychological Differentiation: Studies in Development*, Wiley, New York.

WITKIN, H., DYK, R., FATERSON, H., GOODENOUGH, D. and KARP, S. (1974), *Psychological Differentiation: Studies in Development*, Lawrence Erlbaum, Potomac, Maryland (reprint).

Bibliography

WITKIN, H., GOODENOUGH, D. and KARP, S. (1967), 'Stability of cognitive style from childhood to young adulthood', *Journal of Personality and Social Psychology*, 7, 291–300.

WITRYOL, S. and KAESS, W. (1957), 'Sex differences in social memory tasks', *Journal of Abnormal and Social Psychology*, 54, 343–6.

WOLFF, J. (1972), 'Efficient acoustic parameters for speaker recognition', *Journal of the Acoustical Society of America*, 51, 2044–56.

WOLFF, P. (1963), 'Observation on the early development of smiling', in B. M. Foss (ed.), *Determinants of Infant Behaviour*, II, Wiley, New York.

WOLFF, W. (1933), 'The experimental study of forms of expression', *Character and Personality* 2, 168–76.

WOLFF, W. (1945), *The Expression of Personality*, Harper, New York.

WULF, F. (1922), 'Über die Veränderung von Vorstellungen', *Psychologisch Forschung*, 1, 333–73.

YARBUS, A. (1967), *Eye movement and Vision*, Plenum Press, New York.

YARMEY, D. (1971), 'Recognition memory for familiar public faces: effects of orientation and delay', *Psychonomic Science*, 24, 286–7.

YARMEY, D. (1973), 'I recognize your face but I can't remember your name: further evidence on the "tip of the tongue" phenomenon', *Memory and Cognition*, 1, 287–90.

YARMEY, D. (1974), 'Proactive interference in short-term retention of human faces', *Canadian Journal of Psychology*, 28, 333–8.

YIN, R. (1969), 'Looking at upside-down faces', *Journal of Experimental Psychology*, 81, 141–5.

YIN, R. (1970), 'Face recognition by brain-injured patients: A dissociable ability? *Neuropsychologia*, 8, 395–402.

YOUNG, M. and CAMPBELL, R. (1967), 'Effects of content on talker identification', *Journal of the Acoustical Society of America*, 42, 1250–4.

ZUG, G. (1972), 'A critique of the walk pattern analysis of symmetrical quadrupedal gaits', *Animal Behaviour*, 20, 436–8.

ZUSNE, L. (1970), *Visual Perception of Form*, Academic Press, New York and London.

Name index

Name index

Name index

Subject index

Subject index